Advance praise fo

Fern E.M. Buszowski says that writing about her suffering helped her heal from her suffering. I believe her. These pages hold a strange radiance, a dark crimson glow of deepest wisdom. She writes lucidly and honestly from inside her own pain, and so somehow her story, so deeply personal, becomes our story, too. What's more, she often steps back, gathers a lifetime of accumulated insight about human flourishing, and becomes our teacher and our guide. If you need to embrace life and hope, you've come to the right place.

—Mark Buchanan
author of *God Walk*

With honesty and vulnerability, Fern invites us into her journey, not just of cancer and recovery, but the internal journey of fear and faith, of life and hope. This is so much more than the story of a cancer survivor; these are the reflections of a professional counsellor, a lifelong learner coming alongside us as we walk through the shadows. You'll laugh, you'll cry, and as you engage in the conversations and reflections, you'll grow. It's a must-read for those facing uncertainty and for those of us who imagine we have it all together.

—Rev. Dr. James Paton
Lead Pastor, First Alliance Church

Fern has a beautiful way of using her painful and uninvited journey to bring hope to an unfathomable situation. I love Fern's statement, "A crisis turns life on its head, bringing with it unexpected and unwanted experiences." That says it for each one of us.

And yet Fern's depth of faith and insight brings new life to some age-old truths that we face whenever we are challenged with the unknown. This is a masterful work that takes moments in time to read a bit, ponder a bit, and reshape our thinking a bit, all the while feeling energized by the strength and power that truth has to hold us, to move us forward, and to invite us in to so much more of life. You will be challenged to question your assumptions and you will be given wonderful knowledge and grace to grow and become more of who you were meant to be.

I can't wait to reflectively meander my way through *Embrace Life, Embrace Hope* in a way that will change me and cause me to stretch and become more like Jesus.

Thank you, Fern!

—Ruth Esau
leadership development educator, facilitator, and coach
Urban Pastor with the EMCC

Fern offers us the beautiful gift of being invited into her unexpected journey. Wrapped with raw authenticity, tenacious truth, and practical application, it is a generous gift that glimmers with the hope of Jesus.

—Dr. Rev. Bryce Ashlin-Mayo
Dean of Theology, Ambrose University

As part of Fern's community, I've always been aware of her wisdom and skills as a counsellor, pastor, and spiritual director. I have watched as my beautiful friend Fern has suffered pain and brokenness through her journey with cancer. I had a front row seat to her hard-fought battle to take that head-knowledge and apply it to her own struggles with doubt, anxiety, despair, and grief.

This book bears the marks of her transparency and authenticity in wrestling with God and learning new ways to love Him with all her heart, soul, mind, and strength. Like the kintsugi artists she writes about, her life is even more beautiful today because of the healing and restorative work of God in her heart, soul, mind, and body.

I'm excited to recommend this book to others who are seeking hope and healing.

—Judith Wiebe, spiritual director

This well-written and insightful book by Fern E.M. Buszowski is a must-read for anyone who desires to gain wisdom, knowledge, and understanding. However, I believe even more strongly that it is a must-read for doctors. As a medical practitioner, I have broken bad news and shared serious diagnoses with patients. I have followed their difficult and painful journeys through treatments to save their lives. But I have never actually gone through the journey with them. I have not fully known their inner turmoil, fear, or anxiety as they walked onto the unknown and frightening road of cancer care. I have not followed them home or watched them cry in front of a mirror. I have not journeyed with them behind the closed doors of the radiotherapy suite.

Fern has taken me to those places that I had not been privileged to go with my patients, and I believe everyone, especially healthcare providers, could learn a great deal from the honest details and reflections she shares in this book. She is gracious and appreciative of the high-quality care she received from multiple healthcare workers who dedicatedly provided the care to save her life. Healthcare professionals need to hear these encouraging words because they are people too who often help others through self-sacrifice. Fern's words of encouragement and gratitude are especially meaningful because of her counselling background.

Fern also shares wisdom which I believe we as healthcare workers can learn from to improve on the work that we do. As a physician, for instance, I have asked my patients probing questions without understanding how threatening or even hurtful those questions could be. I have underestimated the especially negative psychological impact a cancer diagnosis (which is often stigmatized) could have on a previously healthy person. Fern reminded me to be better aware of the deeper details and to realize that every second I have could be a useful tool in God's hands.

I consider this book to be a gift to people like me. Fern has graciously invited us into her journey; she has shared intimate and innovative details about finding hope through tremendous challenge. This book is definitely worth reading and sharing with others.

—Dr. Tolu Solola, MD

Embrace Life, Embrace Hope

Cultivating Wholeness and Resilience
through the Unexpected

Embrace Life, Embrace Hope

Fern E.M. Buszowski
MALM, MA Counselling

Editor: Jocelyn A. Drozda
Word Alive Press Editor: Evan Braun

Front Cover Image: Alyssa L. Troung
Back Cover Headshot: Rosalind Coben

Scriptures taken from the Holy Bible, New International Version®, NIV®. Copyright © 1973, 1978, 1984, 2011 by Biblica, Inc.™ Used by permission of Zondervan. All rights reserved worldwide. www.zondervan.com The "NIV" and "New International Version" are trademarks registered in the United States Patent and Trademark Office by Biblica, Inc.™

Disclaimer: While the publisher and author have used their best efforts in preparing this book, they make no representation or warranty with respect to the accuracy or completeness of the contents of this book and specifically disclaim any implied warranties or merchantability or fitness for any particular purpose. No warranty may be created or extended by sales representatives (if any). The advice, perceived advice, insights, and strategies contained in this book may not be suitable for your specific situation. You should consult with a professional where appropriate. Neither the publisher nor author shall be liable for any loss of profit or any other damages but not limited to special, incidental, consequential, or other damages.

While all the stories, anecdotes in this book may be based on real people and experiences the names, locations, and some identifying details, titles, and professions have been altered to protect the privacy of the individuals involved. Any resemblance between these individuals and actual persons is merely coincidental.

Printed in Canada

ISBN: 978-1-4866-2369-3
eBook ISBN: 978-1-4866-2370-9
Hardcover ISBN: 978-1-4866-2371-6

Word Alive Press
119 De Baets Street Winnipeg, MB R2J 3R9
www.wordalivepress.ca

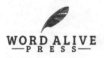

WORD ALIVE
—P R E S S—

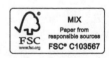

MIX
Paper from
responsible sources
FSC   FSC® C103567
www.fsc.org

Cataloguing in Publication information may be obtained from Library and Archives Canada.

This book is dedicated to my husband Steve:
the love of my life, my encourager, and my supporter
—today, tomorrow, always.

And to my children whose faith and optimism inspire me:
Alyssa and Thich, Becky and Mark. It's a privilege to be your mom.

And to my beautiful grandchildren:
Elliott, Scarlett, Ava, and Lillian. You delight my heart.

I am forever grateful to God for each one of you
and for the hope and insight you instill in me.

Hope means to keep living
amid desperation
and to keep humming
in the darkness.
Hope is knowing that there is love,
it is trust in tomorrow
it is falling asleep
and waking again
when the sun rises.
In the midst of a gale at sea,
it is to discover land.
In the eyes of another
it is to see that you are understood....
As long as there is still hope
There will also be prayer....
And you will be held
in God's hands.[1]
—Henri Nouwen

Contents

Preface

THIS IS WRITTEN FOR you... from my heart to yours. It's a book filled with stories of my experience with oral cancer and some reflections that have produced wisdom and insight in my search for wholeness. Once diagnosed, I journalled with a desire to remember significant moments and make sense of them. I possessed a deep yearning to have a voice and be heard, because at the outset I didn't have any voice at all.

This book encompasses how I tried to cultivate wholeness and find hope while facing a difficult diagnosis of cancer. It's about how my understanding of identity and story tend to intersect and influence how we find hope, meaning, purpose, and wholeness through life's unexpected twists and turns.

To you, my reader, I extend several invitations.

Number one, sit with me as I describe my best recollections of my surgery, treatment, and recovery, all of which taught me lessons and forged deep insight within me. Join me in a firsthand account of my experience of challenges, moments of humour, and the fingerprint of God as He made Himself known to me along the way.

Two, peek into some of my journal reflections as I process and try to make sense of my cancer diagnosis, searching for ways to cope while finding hope and wholeness.

Three, join me in looking through my own integrated lens, which is influenced by my experience of being a counsellor, a retired pastor of counselling and soul care, and a new cancer survivor. Throughout the book I explore my responses to a health crisis while considering new ways to cope and find hope. My training and experience uniquely influence how I take into consideration the needs of my body, soul, and spirit and God's original design for us to be whole.

My deepest desire for you, my reader, is that in my story you can see how I learned, and am still learning, to embrace life, hope, and wholeness—by reflecting on how our human story intimately connects us with God and His story.

There is much contained within these covers. My story and writing are a personal effort and is separate from my profession as a counsellor. At the time of this writing, I was not practicing. In fact, I was preparing for retirement. Now that I've written this book, I'm putting that retirement back on hold.

I'm still learning how to be a cancer patient. I continue to seek out new ways to live well throughout it all. Little did I know that my life would unfold in such a way that everything I knew to be true and held dear would be deeply challenged. Formerly believing myself resilient and strong, always able to bounce back, I found myself needing to develop more resiliency to overcome this new adversity and find new ways of adjusting to my new normal.

As you read, you may find connections to your own story. It's important to write down questions that surface and take the time to reflect on them. If you're anything like me, you might affix a sticky note to the page with your question or take a pencil to jot these questions down in a separate notebook. The moments that raise such questions may be special invitations, golden moments which may benefit you if you give them further consideration. And at the end of each chapter, I have added a summary of its key points, as well as some of my favourite reflection questions that may be helpful.

Whatever crisis you're going through, or if you're caring for someone else in crisis, it's my hope and deepest prayer that you see that hope and wholeness can be found in every journey, even very difficult ones, including your own.

Introduction

MY STORY BEGAN IN 2020 during the pandemic, starting with the surprising diagnosis of oral cancer and followed by a major surgery that rendered me temporarily voiceless. Because visitors were restricted at the time, my only emotional support came through texts from my family. Journalling became a much-needed outlet, giving me a voice for all I experienced.

With so little communication with the outside world, I began writing to my family and those in my closest circle, keeping them updated on my progress and recovery. I started a private blog, which made me feel less alone while isolated in the hospital. In the early days, due to physical limitations, I only wrote a little, yet it came more frequently as I realized that my writing was becoming an avenue to inner healing.

After months of recovery, I decided to write a memoir for my family, my husband, and my children should my life turn out to be a short one—a gift of my heart. This was the birth of my book. As word spread throughout my closest friends, even a year later, every one of them encouraged me to continue and seek publication.

It's my honour and privilege to invite you to join me as I share about my walk toward hope and wholeness and finding ways to live well in my new normal.

ORAL CANCER IS AN invasive, disfiguring cancer that affects its victims in significant ways physically and emotionally for life. Many times, it can kill.

> This year, an estimated 54,000 adults (38,700 men and 15,300 women) in the United States will be diagnosed with oral and oropharyngeal cancer. Worldwide, an estimated 476,125 people were diagnosed with oral and oropharyngeal cancer in 2020.
> Rates of these cancers are more than twice as high in men as in women. White people are slightly more likely to be diagnosed with them than Black people. Oral and oropharyngeal cancer are the eighth most common cancer among men. The average age of diagnosis is 63. About 20% of cases occur in people younger than 55.[2]

Profits from the sale of each book will be donated to cancer research and/or for cancer support programs for cancer patients and families.

Chapter One

CHOICES

You can't get second things by putting them first;
you can get second things only by putting first
things first.[3]

—C.S. Lewis

BLINDED BY BACKGROUND LIGHTS, groggy from medication, I squint, straining to focus on the eyes hiding behind the masked face, his identity concealed further by the glare of the lights behind him. Which one of the three is he? His masked face moves in closer.

As the surgical resident's smiling eyes come into focus, he explains that everything went well. Another surgeon leans in from the other side and shares the same encouraging news.

Vague memories of why I'm here float in and out of my consciousness. *Oh, right. Cancer. Cancer surgery.*

I slip back into a deep sleep.

I awaken, a few hours later, to the *beep-beep-beep* of the machines monitoring my heart and oxygen. A thin transparent tube hangs from a shiny IV pole as condensation collects on the inside of it, silently dripping clear fluid into my arm.

I scan the ICU, trying to get my bearings—and in the process I lift my left hand. *Mum. This is Mum's hand...*

But wait, she's gone. *Mum?*

My awareness continues to clear as I conduct a cursory examination. I can't move. I can't sit up.

I lift my right arm to see where donor skin has been surgically removed to assist in my tongue's reconstruction. The arm, strategically balanced on several pillows to keep it raised, is bandaged wrist to elbow. And here I thought it was going to be a small bandage.

The nurse observes my self-examination and comes close to help me. She reminds me of the operation and gently describes my bandages, the location of my incisions, and informs me why I have a tracheostomy. A tracheostomy means I can't speak at all.

She shows me the whiteboard tucked alongside my bed, which I can use to write on. I motion for the board with my good left hand and write one word: *MIRROR?*

The nurse brings the mirror and holds it up. I cling to her wrist, directing the mirror toward my face and neck. I scan the red, swollen incision along my neck. It extends from below my right ear to the middle of my throat. It's neatly and very evenly stitched closed. Gross, but nicely done. I tell myself it will heal into a wrinkle as I age.

I peer around my face and see a distorted woman looking back. Something is wrong. My face looks lopsided. My reflection shows a puffy face with an ugly, droopy mouth. They warned me about this.

It will recover eventually, I croon internally.

I blink back tears. Two long tubes jut from the Dracula-like holes in my neck. These dangling tubes are attached to my gown by a pin to stop them from pulling as their bulbous ends continuously fill with murky discharge.

I open my mouth and peer inside at the new tongue waiting to greet me. I see a huge, two-toned mass filling my oral cavity. Nothing looks familiar except for my teeth. Part of the tongue looks like mine, but the other part, the new tongue flap, is pinkish white like the skin on my arms. The skin taken from my forearm.

This is not how I imagined it would look. It's smooth-looking but without any taste buds—and it's so swollen that it takes up most of my mouth. The middle of my tongue is no longer in the middle.

I clamp my mouth and eyes simultaneously, unable to bear looking at myself any longer. Not only is it not what I imagined, it's worse.

I want to moan or cry out in horror, but it's impossible. I have no voice. All I can do is cry silent tears as I look into the eyes sadly looking back at me.

I drop my grip on the nurse's arm and she takes the mirror, my hand flopping back onto the pillow. My heart sinks as questions race through my head. How did I not realize this surgery would result in such permanent disfigurement? This isn't me anymore. How am I supposed to live with this? I'll never be the same.

Dread, disgust, and fear invade my heart. Even more questions tumble into my head one after the other. What have I done? Was this a mistake? Is life truly worth living looking like this? With each thought, I sink lower into discouragement.

I ask for the mirror again, but the nurse compassionately and firmly refuses to give it to me. Instead she diverts my attention elsewhere, probably realizing that looking in the mirror won't be helpful in my recovery.

And she's right. It's not profitable for me to dwell on how I look, especially only a few short hours after major surgery.

My husband arrives at the ICU moments later. I hold his hand, with all my might pulling it to my cheek as he leans over and kisses my forehead. The tears flow as I cling to him, voiceless. With his hand against my cheek, I sob inside. I kiss and pat his hand, trying to soothe myself, overcome with emotion. His hand is my lifeline. It infuses me with hope.

Eventually the tears subside, and I find safety and sleep.

When I awake again, I'm struggling to breathe. My tracheostomy is clogged with mucus. Wonderful. More to deal with.

The nurse inserts a suction tube into the tracheostomy to clear the passageway. The suction hurts as it goes in because the tracheostomy plate presses against the raw wound in my throat. It reminds me of the suction hose used during a teeth cleaning—gurgling sounds and all.

Once cleared, air enters more easily into my tracheotomy tube. I take a deep, clean breath. The relief feels good.

Hourly a nurse checks the nerve health of my new tongue flap with a doppler. She presses the wand-like stick gently to my tongue and slowly moves it back and forth until she hears the swish-swish-swish of pulsing blood. My tongue is alive and healthy.

In the morning, nurses prepare to move me to a chair. I wait, my legs hanging over the side of the bed. I feel two leg compression sleeves rhythmically squeeze my legs to help with blood flow and reduce the potential for clots. I peer over the side of the bed as they remove the sleeves and spot a catheter tube leading to a half-filled urine bag alongside the bed.

Ewww. A catheter?

Tubes going in; tubes going out. They're everywhere. Stitches and staples everywhere. There is no swallowing, no fluid, no food. Everything is fed into my body through tubes. Medications and fluids flow through the IV; liquid food moves through the gastrointestinal tube in my nose, reaching deep into my stomach. The catheter? Well, that one helps the fluids exit the body.

Why so many tubes? How can my body heal from all of this?

It seems the only two orifices without tubes are my ears and my butt… and deep inside, I feel a small seed of laughter bubbling up.

It's necessary, I say to myself. *It's temporary.*

Still in the ICU as the disappointment settles in, I wait to be transported to another hospital wing for the remainder of my stay.

As I wait, one nurse waits with me. When the orderly arrives, she leans over to say goodbye. She places her hand on mine and whispers gently, "It was a privilege to care for you. You are beautiful, and you are a very special person. Don't you ever forget that."

A gift of encouragement. Tears well up. These gentle words sear themselves into my heart and fill it with hope as I begin the difficult stages of recovery.

I wonder if God sends us special people like this nurse to bring a much-needed word of hope. I think He does because words of hope tend to stay with you. They are gifts from God.

Hope rises in my heart.

The Influence of Choices

I was unaware that healing is filled with so many interventions, side effects, challenges, setbacks, and pain. And they affect me holistically— physically, mentally, emotionally, and spiritually.

As we face difficult situations, our minds can be like a pendulum rhythmically swinging back and forth from one position to the next. The more it swings, the more you want it to stay still. On the one hand, we desperately want someone or something to take away the pain; on the other, we self-isolate to save ourselves from it. Neither extreme is good. We must determine our locus of control—the location from which we perceive that control of a situation takes place—whether it's outside us or inside us. This affects our perception of a situation. When we uncover our tendencies toward seeing a situation one way or another, we are better able to understand our perspectives and behaviour, allowing us to take the necessary steps to adjust them and be more open to seeing things differently.

I thought about this quite a bit while in the hospital and decided that my locus of control for healing needs to have both internal and external elements. I need both so I can enter a place of wholeness despite the impacts of cancer, surgery, and treatment. Things aren't just being done to me; I can take an active part in the healing process. As an active participant, I have control over how I choose to perceive the circumstances as they unfold.

When a crisis hits, we can feel threatened and react with fear. This is a normal response. But when that fear remains and controls everything we think or do for the long-term, it's unhelpful. I regularly remind myself to remain open and learn to do things differently so I can keep moving forward. I don't measure how fast I move, just *if* I move. Otherwise I'll be stuck in my emotions or lost on some unhelpful tangent.

As a counsellor, I've recommended strategies to help others learn to cope. Now I recommend them to myself—especially the ones that help me face challenging emotions, create new dreams, be grateful, learn, and grow from the opportunities presented.

Change begins with becoming aware of the choices I make, with choosing to listen to the thoughts rolling around in my head, keeping the ones that are helpful and reframing the ones that aren't. I'm choosing to become aware of my emotions and determining where I may need support or help. I'm choosing to embrace a healthy physical lifestyle that enhances my health. I'm choosing to attend to my spiritual needs. I'm being self-compassionate while on this challenging path, making choices that help me rather than hinder me.

All the choices we make in the face of fear impact our healing. We can make choices that move us forward with hope. Our choice of *who* and *what* to trust brings hope along the way. And finding that hope pushes us to survive, even thrive, instead of being solely afraid.

Breathe!

Several days into my hospitalization, I have one such fear-inducing experience. It takes months before I can share it with anyone without breaking down in tears. My perceptions and feelings from the day seem to stick with me, even though I recognize that my memories may be fuzzy.

Early one morning I am being prepared to remove the tracheostomy. The team of three surround me while the resident carefully tells the intern what to do. I can feel the intern gently press on my tracheostomy plate until I hear a *click*. Familiar pain radiates through my still-tender incision.

Some familiar feelings are good, while others aren't.

The intern's eyes widen. "It slipped out!"

"Push it back in."

With another click, the inner tube (called a cannula) snaps into place.

I wish I had a mirror. I can't see anything. What's happening? Maybe it's the same thing they do when cleaning out the tracheostomy tube… it feels similar.

But I can't ask any questions. I still have no voice.

Did it pop out? Partly or the whole thing? What's happening? My mind races, trying to keep up with my imagination, but not as fast as my breath. *Relax. Breathe. Calm down!*

I breathe slowly.

"It's a teaching hospital. You are fine. Everything is fine," the internal counsellor tells me. *"They're learning. The resident has done this hundreds of times. Trust the process. They know what they're doing. Let the intern learn. You were a counselling intern once... people were patient with you as you learned. Be patient. Relax. Breathe."*

I close my eyes and distract myself, allowing their voices to fade into the background.

The whole procedure only takes a few seconds. Then the first resident looks at me and instructs the other resident, "Stay with her!" With that, the other two whisk themselves off to see the next patient.

The remaining resident distracts me from my lightheaded discomfort with interesting stories about why she entered the field of oncology. It isn't long before I feel better and can return to my room. The friendly distraction helped.

Not long after that, I face my next challenge. A small plastic cap called a cork is slipped onto the tracheostomy, allowing me to breathe through my nose and speak. My new task: last twenty-four hours with the cork on, and if successful the tracheostomy can come out.

I try to suck air into my lungs through my mouth and nose. It's like breathing through a bent straw. I can breathe, yes, but it takes a lot of concentration and effort.

But I'm focused on my mission. I want my real voice back.

I have a new oxygen machine with moist air that blows up my nose through two huge prongs resting in my nostrils... nasal passages that haven't been used in many days. I'm not talking about one of those oxygen tubes normally found in hospitals; this one is big, fitting snugly in my nose, secured along my cheeks, and fastened behind my head. It sports a wide hose at the end. The prongs share space in one nostril with the feeding tube while the other rests in the empty nostril in which I have a deviated septum.

It isn't long before the oxygen hurts my nasal passages and my head begins to pound. I grab hold of the air tube and pull the prongs out of my nose. I hold it away while still directing the flow into my nose.

Now what will I do? I can hardly take in enough air to satisfy my lungs. I wonder if this is what suffocation feels like.

My imagination kicks in again and I flash back to when I was a young teen. I relive getting the news that my twenty-three-year-old brother-in-law drowned while kayaking.

Is this what it's like not to be able to breathe? I ask myself. *It must have been terrifying for him.*

I buzz the nurses' station to get help from a respiratory therapist. It feels like hours pass before I ask a second time. I'm desperate, yet they tell me there may be a wait; shift change is coming.

"Try not to think the worst," says the counsellor inside me. *"They're busy. Shift change is coming. Pandemic protocols slow everything down. They're doing the best they can."*

I focus on breathing, all the while feeling abandoned. Fear keeps getting in the way, almost as though it's blocking my breath.

I can't do this.

I almost give up. Tears are my only company.

Then I remember all the breathing exercises I taught others in my practice for so many years. I know they are calming.

Breathe in, breathe out. I count. *Slow it down even more… it makes it easier to breathe. Ten seconds in, ten seconds out.*

I manage to take six slow, agonizing breaths per minute. Am I getting enough oxygen while breathing so slowly? The noisy sounds of my wheezing fill my ears and become a soothing white noise. It takes my mind off my deep discomfort and desire to catch my breath. My chest and stomach move up and down, rising and falling.

Breathe in, breathe out.

Slowly I calm down. The counsellor returns.

"What have you done in the past to help when you're scared or facing something unwanted?" I ask myself.

Trusting God and praising Him despite my circumstances, I answer.

The doxology floats into my mind… a song I learned as a little girl. And so I sing, in my head, *"Praise God from whom all blessings flow…"*

I wonder, why is it that I would only think of God when I'm so desperate? But I keep singing softly in my head, the song distracting me from the stiflingly close air and harsh flow of oxygen. My sense of calm grows as I focus on the goodness of God instead of my discomfort and fear.

Suddenly I feel a gentle rush of peace and gratitude for what I know will help me cope. Craving more, I reach for my tablet, plug in my earphones, and continue to play songs about God's goodness. These songs soothe my heart. I don't have the words to pray, but the songs give me words to remember. They become a sort of prayer.

Time passes like this and calm flows over me despite the effort it takes to breathe.

Shift change.

I buzz and ask again for help from the new nurse. Third time's the charm, they say. The respiratory therapist arrives within minutes and quickly makes a few adjustments.

Relief... finally. Now I can breathe more easily.

Fear

The diagnosis, surgery, and a lengthy hospital stay were the first stages I had to face. And throughout them, many days were filled with fear.

I hate to admit it, but since my diagnosis fear had become the foundation for each new challenge on the road toward healing.

Fear of dying. Fear of living disfigured.

Fear of pain. Fear of suffering.

Fear of choking.

Fear of more needles.

Fear of too much medication. Fear of too little.

Fear of too much radiation. Fear of too little.

Fear of gaining weight. Fear of losing too much weight.

Fear of being a burden.

Fear of exhaustion. Fear of not sleeping well.

Fear of being vulnerable. Fear of not being strong.

Fear of loss. Fear of abandonment.

Fear of being unattractive or unwanted.

Fear of speaking, being misunderstood.

Fear of the cancer reoccurring.

Fear of being embarrassed. Fear of being around others.

Fear of being rejected.

Fear of the unknown.

Fear of more challenges. Fear of being overwhelmed.

Fear of fear itself...

Fear was my companion for months, rearing its ugly head especially when I was at my most vulnerable. Fear is the scary unknown future.

At first, I attributed most of these feelings to the physical overstimulation. When I awakened in the mornings, I felt pain with every single movement. It was my last thought before falling asleep and my first thought upon opening my eyes. There was no relief from the physical sensations; it was relentless and at times I broke down in sheer exhaustion. My exhaustion often stemmed from expending energy to manage the fear.

Emotions can be exhausting.

I finally realized I was fearing that life would never return to normal. It dawned on me that before I could find a way to create a new normal, I had to face the reality of my new and future limitations. I needed to come to terms with a type of normal I could learn to embrace and enjoy given my health. This would be a normal that helped me feel whole.

I began to contemplate what I often explained to my clients about emotions. I had to remind myself of this truth to face my fear.

"We never have to fear fear itself, because it's just an emotion," I would say. *"Our emotions stem from our thoughts. Fear holds no power. If it seems to, it's an unhelpful way of thinking. When we take time to examine our thinking, we can often figure out what we're afraid of and coach ourselves into a new way of thinking. When we find new ways of examining our thinking and bravely face fear, the fear tends to diffuse, to shrink, especially when we explore it and try to make sense of it. As we try to make sense of it, it teaches us that we aren't in control and challenges us to find new ways of trusting God, which can help eliminate the fear."*

Sometimes we can do this alone through reflection, guided imagery, or journalling. Sometimes all we need is a good, safe friend to work through it with us. Sometimes professional help is needed. All are good supports to help us work through how we think so we can learn to make a different choice.

I used every resource available to me to cope through this period.

When we choose to embrace that which makes us fearful and move forward despite it, we enter a place of courage that allows us to keep progressing toward helpful choices. But it's scary to face the thoughts that bring us fear. We just need to take that first step.

We cannot always change our circumstances, but we do have the power to choose how we respond to them. It becomes an opportunity. We can choose courage over fear and become more real and vulnerable by asking for help or encouragement when we need it.

Each struggle we face has purpose, and within each purpose are necessary steps we need to take if we want to figure out how to heal well. It's a process. Healing isn't about the destination. It's about exploring the source of fear. It's about peeling back all the layers, one after the other, and discovering freedom from fear.

With each challenge we face, as we learn to examine our perceptions and beliefs about the impact of these experiences, we become more resilient and find new and better ways to cope.

Each challenge does bring with it an opportunity, but we must diligently search for it. We tend to look only at the source of the crisis and its impact—and react with fear. We often forget to look ahead to how that challenge can transform us into better and stronger people. Cultivating this type of mindset can help us see opportunities and welcome hope.

We always tell ourselves stories about our experiences. Let's choose stories that bring us hope.

Some of the choices we make bring life to our soul while others bring death. By knowing the difference between the two, we can cautiously guard our hearts and minds to live well with the time we are given on this earth. But there are no guarantees... just opportunities and choices.

Fear can motivate, and fear can cripple. It's what we do with fear that counts.

> **Some of the choices we make bring life to our soul while others bring death.**

Why Me?

A few days after my release from the hospital, my surgeon reviews the results of my pathology report. I still don't have an answer to my original question: why do I have cancer? If we don't know why, what is the prognosis? What's the chance of the cancer returning? That's the question that plagues me.

The tumour the doctors removed during surgery was larger than first estimated. Thankfully, no cancer was found in the lymph nodes. That's the good news. The bad news? Evidence was found of the cancer trying to reach a nerve so it could spread through my body.

Surgery alone wasn't enough. Radiation treatment is recommended.

Tears flow in a mix of confusion. I feel some relief from the good news, but dread also arises from the bad news and my unknown future.

I decide to find a way to learn to live without knowing all the answers, to trust the process and choose the recommended radiation treatment. I choose not to focus on the statistical risks of side effects, because more good than bad will come from the treatments. Instead I choose to trust the process, trust my doctors, and trust God. After all, my life is in their hands anyway.

Except when I keep forgetting to trust. That's when fear slips back in.

Trust Found in Not Knowing

The challenging thing about going through a crisis, as a counsellor, is that most often I know what's good for me and what isn't. I joke about my inner thoughts and self-coaching habits. My training is so ingrained in me that I can't get away with developing unhelpful habits of mind, because I deeply desire authenticity—inside and out.

The counsellor mindset is there all the time, monitoring and reminding me to choose well at every emotional and mental turn. To keep the counsellor happy, I've learned to cultivate self-compassion—acknowledging the difficulty of the situation, demonstrating empathy, being kind to myself, and giving myself permission to ask for help when needed (and to take it when offered).

I have learned to coach myself when I see myself going down the wrong road. I tell myself, *"It's okay not knowing—not knowing why I ended up with cancer, not knowing what my outcome will be. And it's okay to be uncomfortable with the not knowing. It's okay to be vulnerable. You are only human. Just because you're a counsellor doesn't mean you can't hurt, be afraid, or become overwhelmed. Your reactions are normal. This was major surgery. There is disfigurement, pain, and tightness. Life has changed. You are different. Yet change and being different isn't necessarily bad. Remember to take the opportunity to look for the good."*

Not knowing forces me to move from falsely believing I have complete control over a situation to learning that I can only control my responses and choose to trust God more, trust my team of doctors to care for me and manage my health, and trust myself to reach out to others for support when needed.

Cultivating trust in our relationships builds a safety net and helps us grow, learn, and gain new perspectives and insights, even when we face big challenges. Best of all, it helps to diffuse fear. But it requires us to be vigilant about what's going on inside us and be vulnerable enough to acknowledge it when it's unhelpful—and change if necessary.

Focusing my mind and thoughts on what brings life and love helps me cultivate gratitude so that I appreciate what I have instead of resenting what I don't, or what I've lost, or in comparing my life to others' seemingly pleasant lives.

Managing Expectations

It's important to face and accept the reality of our circumstances. It's equally important to lament the losses, acknowledge the impacts, and grieve. This is a healthy balance. Doing only one or the other creates an imbalance—or worse, it can keep us stuck or looking for answers that misdirect us and prevent us from moving forward.

Like everyone else, my expectations are influenced by my past, present, and dreams of my future. How tightly I choose to hold onto these expectations, seeing them as the only way to experience life, will affect what happens when things *don't* turn out as expected. A crisis turns life on its head, bringing with it unwanted experiences.

When I rigidly believe that my life needs to go a certain way, I'll struggle more in the face of the unanticipated. Then all my energy gets tied up in anger and resentment instead of healing. Hanging on too tightly to expectations keeps me stuck, and in the end it often causes more pain, wasting valuable time better spent on cultivating wholeness in my life.

My experience with cancer has reminded me that nothing on this earth is truly permanent. Learning to discard all my fixed expectations about how life should go helps me remain open to new experiences. I'm then better able to adapt to changing environments, conditions, and yes, even suffering. Life has many good qualities, but it also has difficult ones. We can experience loss, suffering, and tragedy. When I expect both the good and the difficult, I'm not shocked when they come.

Reflecting on these challenges and coping mechanisms, I realized that I hadn't asked any *what* or *how* questions, which may have been more helpful in moving forward, because I had wasted so much time asking *why* questions about the past.

I could have asked questions like these. What do I need to do to help myself deal with this? What will help me? Despite these circumstances, what do I have to be grateful for? How will this change my life for good even though it's difficult to experience? How can I not feel so alone or abandoned in this? What opportunities are being presented to me in this moment? How will God use this to grow me into a better version of myself? In what way has God been more present to me through this experience?

As I reflect on the answers to these questions, they bring about a new openness in my heart, helping me to choose and embrace hope as I step even closer toward accepting my circumstances.

> **...most times we can't change our circumstances. But we can change how we choose to perceive and think about them.**

Looking for the Opportunity

We can't always control our environment, and most times we can't change our circumstances. But we can change how we choose to perceive and think about them. When we expand our *why* questions to include other types of inquiry about the present and future, we can go from being a victim to being a survivor—a survivor with purpose.

Being a survivor doesn't mean we will never be scared or will only feel strong inside all the time. It's about acknowledging current reality while taking small steps moving forward with hope and courage. It's about believing that God's mercy is available, that He is present and still a good God even during hard and unwanted circumstances. It's about believing we are never alone, crisis or not.

Sean Campbell of the ministry Samaritan's Purse has seen much tragedy, crises, and loss throughout his career. He says,

> When are you and I closest to God? Not when times are good, but when times are tough. Because it's in times like that the mercy of God is extended to us, and we sense that. His mercy is always extended to us, but we just sense it in a greater way when times are tough.[4]

It's the kind of mercy that invites us to believe in hope. It causes us to believe He is there with us, especially when others aren't. It doesn't mean He will take away all our difficulties or pain, but He is with us every step of the way. That belief, that trust, is the hope that accompanies us, often helping us to embrace a new type of wholeness. The hope helps me to see opportunities and become more resilient in choosing to live well right now where I'm at.

Seeing my surgical incisions and new tongue in the mirror marked the very beginning of my healing. I needed to see the new me—the surgically altered me—to understand what changes were necessary for me to survive, thrive, and discover the new reality I needed to embrace.

Since then, I've had to accept several more realities and find ways to release their associated fears. It's the difficult realities, the ones with us presently with all their limitations and challenges, that we need to accept first. In many ways, these are invitations to receive gifts that release us from fear.

There is no perfect time to start. But we do need to start. With faith, trust, and by making wise choices, we can hold on to the hope that maybe, somehow, the future will be even better than what we had before.

HIGHLIGHTS

The challenge is in the choices we make that bring us life. We must choose to live well now, in the present, with joy and hope, despite the unknown.

Reflections

Consider What Keeps Us Stuck

- Fear is a normal response to dangerous things such as a scary, unknown future. When fear controls everything we think or do in the long-term, it's unhelpful in helping us to achieve healing. It's what we do with fear that counts.

Consider What Brings Life

- All the choices before us will make a difference in our healing.
- We cannot always change our circumstances, but we do have the power to choose how we respond to them.
- Each challenge brings with it an opportunity and a gift, but we must diligently search for them.
- Cultivating trust in our relationships builds a safety net, helping us to grow, learn, and gain new perspective and insights, even when the road is challenging.
- We strike a healthy balance when we lament our losses, acknowledge their impacts, and grieve while accepting the reality of our situation.

Personal Reflection

- What is one thing you could start doing that would bring some life, peace, laughter, and contentment? For example, go for a walk, read a good book, invite a friend for coffee, listen to music, take a class, or join a support group.

- Check how often your mind wanders to the past or the future and whatever it is you're thinking about.
- What is one worry or fear you find yourself dwelling on that makes you feel stuck? If your best friend had this same fear, what words of encouragement would you give to help them to cope better?

Chapter Two

EXPECTATIONS

Remember that emotion is not a debatable phenomenon. It is an authentic reflection of our subjective experience, one that is best served by attending to it.[5]

—Curt Thompson, MD

SQUEAK-SQUEAK. MY BED sighs as my muscles strain to find comfort in the high-tech hospital bed. I miss my bed at home. I want my husband and kids. Here, I have no family, no friends, and no visitors.

No relief.

I'm bone weary and sorely alone. It's worse than any pain I've experienced before because it's a heart pain, one that can't be measured or monitored.

I'm usually alone when unwanted questions come visiting—similar yet worded differently each time, sometimes gently, never unkindly, but sometimes directly.

"Do you smoke?" someone asks.

I can only nod or shake my head when people talk to me. But I wish I could voice what I'm really thinking.

I don't smoke but did experiment as a teenager for a few years. My dad smoked while I was growing up. Could that be the reason for developing cancer?

"So… not a smoker. Do you drink?"

Drink? You mean alcohol? As a teen I experimented, and into my early twenties when we'd go out for supper and dancing, but not since then. I might have six glasses of wine per year, if that. Sometimes years go by without me having any wine—I prefer bubbly, flavoured water, good food, and chocolate... lots of it! For some reason, drinking wine makes my toes ache so I normally keep away from it except on rare occasions... I do make my own vanilla flavouring with vanilla beans soaked in vodka. Could that be the cause? But I only use a teaspoon of it in my baking, and only if it's called for in a recipe.

"No? Not that either."

My chest tightens as the tagteam of indignation and defensiveness come at me. How am I supposed to respond? My tight muscles feel exhausted deep inside my chest. With each additional question, my defences are further worn down...

The counsellor mindset drowns out my fears. She's back to coach me, telling me to breathe and let it go. *"You're feeling shame and shame never tells the truth. This list of questions is only about identifying risk factors, not causes for your cancer. Now breathe."*

I sink back into the soft bed and wait until the questions are over.

With time, I choose curiosity. But my curiosity is tainted with a little of my own judgment. What ever happened to open-ended questions? What about giving someone the benefit of the doubt? There are always exceptions to the main causes of cancer.

I remind myself about the nice surgical resident who mentioned that sometimes older adults whose dentures rub repeatedly on existing sores can develop oral cancer. At night, my tongue *did* rub against my rough-edged retainer. It was the exact same spot where the sore had developed. So maybe that was the cause.

But we really don't know.

My head pounds. My forehead aches. My eyes sting from sleep deprivation. This must be what it feels like to be hit by a train. The discomfort forces my filter to lower an inch more. I feel vulnerable and weak, invaded, poked, measured, and monitored every hour or two.

"Breathe," the counsellor tells me. *"Be careful what you choose to believe about their words. Shame only sticks when we let it. They're just asking questions to learn your history. You know that. Focus on the fact that*

they're trying to help. They probably don't realize how these questions affect you."

Hours later, there's another shift change. New people. More questions.

I catch myself thinking an unhelpful *Here we go again!* I wonder how I can better prepare to coach myself each time such questions come. "*These are good, kind people. They're only trying to help you. Focus on the good.*"

The first few times, I fail miserably. I immediately feel the shame arriving with the questions. I'm surprised how long it lingers afterward. But eventually I remember to ask myself my own questions to distract myself when I sense shame creeping into my heart.

What's going on in my body? What shame messages am I receiving? What's the first thing I said to myself when I felt shame show up? What's underneath the shame? Am I mind-reading when I think I understand their motives? Am I jumping to a conclusion? Is there any truth to what they're saying? What am I saying to myself that isn't helpful?

Shame tends to sneak up on me. I wish there was another way to process this stuff. I close my eyes and begin.

It's your image you care about. The words float into my head. *Really? My image is at stake?*

I think about how privileged and proud I am about having served in charities, ministries, and educational systems throughout most of my career. Indignantly, I admit that I probably care way too much about what others think of me. I want to be seen as kind, compassionate, a helpful contributor to society. And maybe even a little purehearted too. And I want to be seen as someone with integrity. I want to be authentic, the same me inside as the me outside, with no contradictions between what I say and what I do.

Other people's words can feel unjust, like an unwanted identity pushed on me. No one sees the real me, just the false identity that shame imposes. Too often I let others' words shame me when maybe it's not even their intent.

The counsellor shows up again. I really wish she'd go help someone else.

Am I overthinking it? Am I telling myself an untrue story? I just assume that I know other people's motives. The counsellor reminds me, though, that others may just be curious too. It's easy for non-specialists, or others in related fields, to misconstrue risk factors and causes. It's important to listen to what your doctor tells you, not the others.

So once again I choose to extend the benefit of the doubt.

Early on, unexpected questions and comments, and my reactions to them, weakened my resolve to persevere and recover. I had to work hard at learning to step back out and move into curiosity instead of judgment.

I needed to hear something helpful, perhaps something empathetic and encouraging like "It must be hard not knowing why this happened to you. You're doing well. Keep on doing what you're doing. We'll help you along the way."

Those words would have given me hope.

Labels

How we respond to others communicates to them who we think they are, one way or another, through body language, words, eye contact, and tone of voice. Are we open and welcoming or do we employ words and behaviours that make others feel shamed or unwelcome? What do we want to be known for? Being welcoming or unwelcoming? Shaming or encouraging? It all stems from how we think and judge people, and through these thoughts and judgments we relay whether another person is loved, accepted, or valued. In some cases, these people are fighting just to stay alive.

We will all experience unhelpful comments at one point or another. How we respond will make a big difference. When we choose to respond with patience, curiosity, and love, we can help others understand the impact of their words. In this way, we model the kind of loving behaviour we prefer to receive. If we want others to be sensitive to our feelings, we need to extend the same courtesy to them.

When we judge other people's words as being "unkind" or "mean," as I did, we jump to a conclusion, believing that we know their motives.

In so doing, we assign them a label and fail to see that they may just be trying to help.

When this happens, we see ourselves as victims and them as perpetrators. When we take on the identity of the victim, we often want someone to rescue us. Then a third person is needed, someone with whom we can complain, vent, or gossip about the situation. This only entrenches our perspective even further—and in the end we really don't know other people's motives.

Moreover, we don't have to accept anyone's ideas as our own. Friends, family, and caregivers aren't uncaring because they're ignorant about our experience or unaware of the impact of their words. They're human and are learning to understand or cope with a difficult situation. In most cases, they don't know what to say or do to help us feel better.

On days when we feel unseen or unjustly labelled, we need to build a better understanding of our own identity. This will help us process such moments in ways that are helpful.

Who Am I? Whose Am I?

Understanding our own identity will help us build resiliency against other people's judgments or false beliefs. Acknowledging that others have identities too can help us choose wise and healthy expectations in our relationships.

We all define our identity in different ways. Sometimes we use career titles, status, and income. Or maybe we're influenced by our talents, interests, educational background, grades, family, culture, faith, gender, privilege, social status, financial status, and opportunity. These factors can provide insight into what, where, when, and how we make a living.

But they don't get to the heart of one important question, one that's rarely asked which is the foundation to all the others. It's the question of our authentic identity: *who am I?*

We can't answer this question without posing another important question: *whose am I?*

Finding answers to these two questions leads us to better understand our identity, our value, and our purpose. These answers influence our response and our ability to be resilient in a crisis.

Identity Expectations

When we face a crisis, our belief regarding our identity is challenged—sometimes more deeply than we would like. We might ask ourselves, *Why me? What have I done to deserve this? Am I being punished for something? What does this say about me?* Understanding and accepting our identity starts with how we think about ourselves.

We aren't what we face, what we do, what others do to us, what they think about us or say to us. This is the manifestation of shame. The crises we experience don't define us. However, they can give us the opportunity to learn more about who we are, and Whose we are, so we can heal, grow, and mature with a broader, clearer perspective of our value.

> **The crises we experience don't define us. However, they can give us the opportunity to learn more about who we are, and Whose we are...**

As we take the time to examine our beliefs, we will be faced with having to decide whether the image we believe to be our identity is, in fact, true at all, or whether it's a fabricated, false identity.

If our identity is deeply grounded in who God is, then it's separate from our circumstances. It can be challenging to believe that our identity and circumstances are separate from each other when difficult circumstances arise, because we tend to want to judge and assign blame. When we know our identity and inherent value, we can remind ourselves that our identity doesn't come from external factors like what happens to us or what others say, do, or think about us.

For me, the identity question started early in my life. But every time I thought I had the answer, it was as though someone came along and snatched it away. For some reason, I believed that I needed approval, to be authenticated by someone wiser and more powerful than me, whether it be a parent, older sibling, authority figure, or employer. I could never stand firm long enough to see whether my identity was the real me. The search continued for years.

Being the youngest child of an engineer and a nurse, there was an expectation that my siblings and I would excel in math and the sciences. My brothers and sister were also more athletic, intelligent, and mathematically and scientifically gifted than me. I was more interested in recreation, art, ideas, languages, stories, and people. It took a long time for me to figure out that we had different but equally valuable interests and talents.

Instead I learned to not draw undue attention to myself. Flying under the radar was the best course of action, because I knew that I wouldn't be noticed if I could be seen as quiet and obedient—basically invisible. This gave me the freedom I valued.

Leaning into such a false belief means that we live to please others. It blinds us to truths about ourselves and shuts down our authentic identity. We are no longer our authentic selves but rather a version of ourselves others want us to be. It's a version of ourselves adjusted for others to accept us.

When we're little, we often take on behaviours for survival purposes. It doesn't have to be a life-or-death situation for this to occur; it can just be to make us feel safe and secure. The ability to remain under the radar served me well until I became an adult. But when we age, these learned behaviours catch up with us. They may have been helpful as coping mechanisms when we were young, but they become unhelpful and inhibiting as adults.

As I grew into adulthood, my identity became clearer each year, yet my voice didn't always line up with who I thought myself to be. There were still contradictions.

But I never recognized them. I became lost in trying to find my way through early adulthood. I spent the first ten years of my career in the IT world climbing the corporate ladder. At thirty-seven years of age, I was responsible for a team of twenty-four systems engineers, traveling weekly between two large cities after an international corporate takeover. It was exciting but exhausting.

The money was amazing, but my heart longed for home. I had young children at home, and all I wanted was to be with them. But because I believed that I had to prove my own value to myself, I used status and income as a measuring tool to define my value.

Finally, one night, alone in a hotel, while reading and reflecting on my life, tearful and lonely, I decided that I needed to resign even though our family income would drop by sixty percent.

That alone time in the hotel helped me clear enough room in my head and heart to make a decision that was right for me and my family. Not only did it help me realize what I needed to do, but it also helped me learn about who I am and Whose I am.

The realization was sparked by a guidebook that went with a Bible study I was taking at my church. The books came with me back and forth on the plane; I spent my nights studying, learning, and growing spiritually. We had moved west the year earlier and had decided it was important to incorporate faith into our children's upbringing, so we had begun attending church. Little had I known how much this decision would alter the course of my life.

At church I learned about my authentic identity from God's perspective—not anyone else's and certainly not my own misguided, culturally popular understanding. I learned that all humans are made in God's image. We are designed to be whole. We are physical, emotional, spiritual, and psychological beings. We have value because of who He is, not because of anything we do, where we come from, or how much money, education, or status we have.

It is life-changing to understand that God ultimately created us, and that we are of great value. This changed my perceptions. It changed me. It changed my life.

Knowing that God created every human with great value, as an act of love, is something I can trust. He does this for every single person on this earth. I'm not the only one who's special; everyone is. Everyone is loved and has a purpose. Everyone. When I learned this, my perspective and attitude about myself and others changed.

Only when I was able to combine this new truth with knowing how I was wired psychologically, as well as spiritually, could I begin to glimpse my true self. Along with this, a deep sense of freedom followed. Recognizing my identity, talents, and abilities, even with all my limitations, was incredibly freeing… whereas trying to earn my value by doing things was exhausting.

Unwanted life experiences often produce a crisis of faith and cause us to question our identity. All the crises I've gone through so far in my life have impacted how I see myself. Or maybe, as I've come to learn, they were just opportunities for me to gain greater clarity about who I am.

When I learned about my identity and value, it became the foundation upon which I could process and make sense of my life today. It has become the steppingstone I use to face difficult situations and recover with hope, even when facing a disfiguring diagnosis such as oral cancer.

Sometimes I forget. When I remember and reset my focus, my perspective changes, my faith and trust grow, my gratitude comes, and hope fills my heart.

Attachments

A solely secular view of our identity, or how we come to believe who we are, is influenced by our experiences through our attachments, parenting, upbringing, and relationships with others. Yet there is a missing piece: a spiritual view. Add this to the secular view of our identity and we gain a more inclusive perspective. When it comes to secular and spiritual, it's not either/or but both/and.

Attachment theory, often studied by counsellors, describes an infant's need for proximity to their primary caregivers for emotional security and survival. A child will use their caregiver as a secure base from which to explore and return to for safety and support in times of perceived threat or danger.[6] These early relationships with our caregivers affect our future attachment styles throughout life.

We have imperfect relationships because we are imperfectly human. Therefore, the attachment styles we've developed may not always be secure; they can affect how we see ourselves, others, and even God.

The good news is that they can change over time in healthy, safe relationships.

From a spiritual view of identity, author David Benner writes about how important it is for us to know how God sees us, because it affects how we will relate to Him and others.[7] Do our attachment styles influence how we see God? How we believe God sees us? Will we dismiss or ignore God, or be overly obedient and legalistic due to a deep fear of being rejected?

Or will we offer ourselves humbly and vulnerably to a safe God who loves us no matter what? Will we try to earn His approval by doing more, by doing good, by doing better like we do for our human parents? Our typical ways of thinking about who God is, how we relate to Him, and how He might see us is often dualistic. Maybe we need to take some time to contemplate how we see Him.

In *Falling Upward,* author Richard Rhor describes "a newly discovered capacity for what many religions have called 'non dualistic thinking' or both-and thinking."[8] We often think dualistically. We tend to think only secularly or spiritually, right or wrong, one thing and not the other. This approach is often based in comparison. Cultivating a more contemplative way of seeing things "grows almost unconsciously over many years of conflict, confusion, healing, broadening, loving, and forgiving reality. It emerges gradually as we learn to 'incorporate the negative,' learn from what we used to exclude…"[9]

This requires the ability to embrace the mystery of not knowing everything for sure and instead become open to look at God, His purposes, and His ways as a whole. We don't need to do anything to earn God's love. We don't need to adjust ourselves to be acceptable. We just need to be authentically us, because we're good enough for God. He works with us just as we are.

Being confident in God's love and resting securely in it affects how we see ourselves, how we see God, and how we see others. It even influences how we see and experience our circumstances, providing a helpful foundation from which we can make some sense or meaning from our experiences.

Emptying the Clutter

Busy schedules, competing agendas, worries, and stress all contribute to keeping my mind full of clutter. By clutter, I mean my own expectations which keep me distracted and anxious about my circumstances.

The one thing that helps me most in my search for clarity about my identity is to pray and be quiet. I take regular time to pray, giving me opportunities for the normally hidden questions stored in my heart to come to mind. Then I can empty out the clutter in my heart, explore unhelpful expectations I'm hanging onto that which keeps me stuck, and make room for what God has for me to see or hear.

If you're anything like me, you often expect life to play out in a certain way. This leads us to believe that our expectations are the only way in which something can occur. This is more of the same kind of dualistic type thinking we discussed earlier. We think we know what's right and true. It's almost as if when things go wrong, someone has made a mistake. We feel like a victim and believe it's just not fair.

What helps me evaluate my situation is to cultivate curiosity and use a series of questions I call the ladder of expectation. The questions below follow this process:

- What are my expectations in this situation?
- Is this an expectation of something I believe I deserve or have a right to? Is there a hint of pride in believing that I am right about this, or do I somehow believe I am entitled to these expectations?
- By not obtaining what I expect, do I feel devalued or shamed? And have I moved to judgment or blame against someone or something, becoming unwilling to see other points of view because I think I know what is best?
- How long have I been in this place of judgment? Has my behaviour resulted in a lack of forgiveness toward others, myself, or God? Do I feel like a victim because of the situation? Who am I judging or blaming? What unhelpful part am I playing in this?

- Have I moved past unforgiving attitudes whereby the offence festers? Am I acting with resentment or showing contempt toward others, God, or myself?
- Am I beginning to self-isolate from others, protecting myself because I think no one else understands what I'm going through?
- Worse yet, is all of this moving me away from God or making me avoid spending quiet time with Him?[10]

These questions help me to see the false expectations that are driving my life. It gives me a chance to cultivate curiosity and change my thinking to create new and more realistic expectations.

When we embrace false expectations, we tend to compile a list of what's good or bad...

When we embrace false expectations, we tend to compile a list of what's good or bad in the current circumstances. That's a dualistic way of seeing things and it can define what or who we judge to be good for bad for us.

A life of dualistic expectations is a life that revolves around our own perceived needs and desires. It often leads to behaviours that seek to protect us from all the things we may perceive as bad. This gives us a decidedly inward focus and keeps us rigidly fixed in our perspectives.

It's exhausting.

When we live this way, we no longer enjoy the freedom of choice because we are bound by our expectations. We live protectively and life becomes little more than a scoreboard on which we tally all the wins and losses we experience.

Often we lose—and when we lose, we self-isolate to protect ourselves. We lose even more when we withdraw from others.

We do this with people, intentionally avoiding them. It's subtle at first, but then it becomes targeted. Next we may try hiding from God and even blame Him for all that may not be right in our world. We raise the walls higher to protect ourselves even more, believing that we need to do things on our own—after all, don't we know best? We pull away from Him, His teachings, and His purposes, thinking that we're in control and know better. We can pull away from God just enough to distance ourselves yet feel comfortable enough in calling ourselves a person of faith.

The last act of self-isolation, and the saddest, is when we distance ourselves from ourselves. We stop seeing our world accurately. We stop processing our experiences because they are overwhelming. We become dismissive, avoidant, angry, self-shaming, and other-shaming. We distract, become numb, keep busy, reach for unhelpful substances, and indulge in unhealthy activities from technology to gossiping, overeating, overworking, overmedicating, etc.

These coping behaviours push us to a place where we no longer reflect on our experiences but react to them, or even totally ignore them. This shows up in our inner dialogue and behaviours toward others. It may show up through judgment, criticism, unforgiveness, resentment, testiness, and anger.

We tend to compare our experiences with everyone else's and wonder why our world looks so bleak. We wonder why we don't have what we think we deserve. We see ourselves as targets because of the way others behave toward us—or we see ourselves as victims of our own circumstances. Our world shrinks and our pain becomes like an insatiable rogue we nurture and feed. In short, we become lost. Stuck.

Recognizing our own unhelpful behaviour gives us the opportunity to change direction at any point. This recognition can help us to keep moving forward, toward people and toward God.

True Belonging

Many years ago, I began taking part in a simple exercise that started me along my search to better understand my own identity. Here's how it started for me.

I slip into an empty chair at a morning ladies retreat, looking around the room for some familiar faces. The leader invites us to quiet our hearts. I take three slow, deep breaths and feel my stress and concerns melt away. Now I'm present.

The leader is a registered nurse in the mental health ward at a nearby hospital. She can integrate science and faith particularly well. She's also a bubbly, active volunteer at our church.

She introduces a guided prayer time which she calls meditation. Opening her Bible, she turns to Psalm 63 and with quiet confidence rhythmically reads the passage, pausing for emphasis which helps the words penetrate my heart. Scripture is a beautiful foundation for reflection and a welcomed invitation to learn and draw close.

> *You, God, are my God, earnestly I seek you; I thirst for you, my whole being longs for you, in a dry and parched land where there is no water. I have seen you in the sanctuary and beheld your power and your glory. Because your love is better than life, my lips will glorify you. I will praise you as long as I live, and in your name I will lift up my hands. I will be fully satisfied as with the richest of foods; with singing lips my mouth will praise you.* (Psalm 63:1–5)

She reads and rereads the passage, each time adding a different emphasis.

Slowly, she guides the meditation: "Imagine yourself walking through your home, along the hallway toward your bathroom. You open the door and steam pours out. Imagine the bathroom mirror is all steamed up from someone taking a hot shower."

She pauses to give us time to form this image in our imaginations. Silence envelops the room.

"Now imagine that God's hand reaches down and begins to write something on the steamy mirror. He writes a special word or note just for you. Watch as He prints each letter on the mirror. Then lean in and see what He wrote."

I close my eyes, relax, and allow these images to come to mind. I'm a visual person and my imagination engages. Guided imagery is a technique we often use in counselling, but at this time in my life I had never used it with Scripture. This was a first for me.

I see myself walk down the hallway and open the bathroom door as steam floats out. As it dissipates, an extended index finger reaches out from behind the steam, tracing letters on the fogged-up mirror. I lean forward and strain to read the letters.

YOU ARE MINE. I AM YOURS. I LOVE YOU!

My heart lurches in my chest. Those words—*YOU ARE MINE*—hit me deeply.

I am His? God is mine? A new awareness fills my mind. *Our relationship is two-way! It's reciprocal. He is the one I love most, and out of this love must flow my life, my relationships, and my responses to life.*

The leader tells us to take some quiet time to reflect on what is coming to mind. I journal and rest with these thoughts and wonder. If this is true, then He must value me.

I belong to God. I am good enough.

When we move toward God and toward people, developing a deep sense of belonging, we learn more about our identity, worth, and purpose. In the process, we gain new meaning along the way, no matter what comes.

HIGHLIGHTS

Knowing our own identity helps us to build resiliency against others' judgment or false beliefs. Developing a clear understanding of our identity influences how we form and process our expectations to keep us moving forward toward others and toward God. Acknowledging that others have an identity too can help us choose wisely and form healthy expectations surrounding our relationships.

Reflections

Consider What Keeps Us Stuck

- Become aware and release any untrue or made-up stories in which we magically know another person's motives when we don't really know at all.
- Examine any unhelpful expectations that can label, blame, or shame ourselves or others.

Consider What Brings Life

- Cultivate curiosity, explore our true identity and its source, and understand our unique value.
- Manage our expectations so we can move from disappointment and judgment to acceptance and forgiveness.

Personal Reflection

- Think of an expectation you hold that has not been met. Reflect on it using some of the questions outlined in the ladder of expectation. Add some of your own questions. Journal any impressions that come to mind. Consider your answers. What is one thing you might do that could change the way you look at things? Journal your reflections.

Chapter Three

WHOLENESS

Owning our story and loving ourselves through that
process is the bravest thing that we will ever do.[11]

—Brené Brown

THE CRISES WE FACE often bring unwanted chapters into our lives. When we slow down to read these difficult chapters, we gain new insights that can enrich our lives.

> **One, we are designed to heal. Two, sometimes healing hurts. The hurting doesn't mean you aren't healing.**

I learned two profound things, both from my surgeon, during my recovery. One, we are designed to heal. Two, sometimes healing hurts. The hurting doesn't mean you aren't healing.

Designed for Healing

I watch in awe how the four surgical sites on my body—arm, leg, neck, and tongue—slowly heal and transform. My surgeon gently cleans the thick scabs from my arm. I feel nothing but numbness, unless numbness is a feeling.

"This will help it heal better," he says.

I comment, "I'm amazed how the body heals. It's kind of neat to watch."

He listens as he continues to examine the donor site on my arm where the surgical team removed a flap of skin and a long nerve to reconstruct my tongue. A thin layer of skin shaven from my upper thigh was then used to do a skin graft, allowing new skin growth to repair the donor site on my arm.

"Your body," he says, "was designed that way."

His words hang in the silence. A new thought rolls into my mind: *How I am today does not mean I'll be this way tomorrow.* The words enter my heart, bringing a small glimmer of hope.

These few simple words, stated with assurance and confidence, are profoundly encouraging to me—even now, many months later. They give me hope and push out any discouragement that seeps in.

We are designed to heal.

> **God made us to be whole—that's part of His story for us.**

I know this to be true physically because healing is happening right before my eyes. But after some reflection on what it means to heal, I am equally confident that this is true emotionally and spiritually.

We are designed to heal. We are designed to be whole.

God made us to be whole—that's part of His story for us. This is the original plan for mankind: to heal and to be whole.

In moments when we're hurting, suffering, or confused, I wonder whether the deep longings for wholeness might be God wooing us to Himself, inviting us into the healing journey that is His story for us.

Designed for Wholeness

What does this mean for me? What does it mean for you?

If God designed us to be whole, and we aren't whole—not fully, not yet—how can the perspectives we hold about our messy or hard stories help us move toward wholeness and healing?

We use words like "I'm processing" or "I'm working through things," as though we only start the search for healing and wholeness once we recognize that something is broken and we expect to get it fixed. Or worse, we expect things to return to the way they were before they were broken.

But becoming whole doesn't mean getting fixed or going back to life as it was. That's impossible. It's impossible because every crisis changes us. We can't be the same person we once were. If we could, we'd need to unlearn and ungrow from all we previously experienced and learned.

Our expectations influence how we interpret, process, and respond to our unfolding story. When we don't get what we expect, we can expend a lot of energy thinking about how to change things. This turns us into complainers who feel resentful, angry, stuck... exhausted.

In situations when we can't influence or change the circumstances outside of our control, our unfulfilled expectations can impact our behaviour even if we aren't aware of them. When we stubbornly desire our expectations to be met, it's more difficult to accept our circumstances when the unexpected happens. Developing an awareness of the expectations that hold us back from accepting uncontrollable experiences helps us to gain new skills to refocus, learn, grow, and move toward healing and wholeness instead of staying stuck.

When difficult times enter our lives, knowing our identity, what we believe, and in what, where, and whom we place our faith and hope will help in the process of welcoming wholeness—the kind of wholeness that integrates body, mind, and spirit. A wholeness that brings peace and hope.

Ann Voskamp, a Canadian author, writes that many of us can become stuck in the middle of our story. She says that the story isn't over. If our story isn't over, we aren't at the end of it yet, because His stories have always worked out. God hasn't forgotten us.

As I read her words, I think about it. I don't know the future or what it holds, but it's true that His stories have always worked out. Maybe mine will too. This is a good thought.

Voskamp writes,

> You haven't forgotten us or this chapter or this story, and if You haven't forgotten us, we're not about to go forgetting that Your stories always work out in the end—and if things aren't working out quite yet, it just means we're not quite yet to the end. We'll literally practice our faith—we'll practice saying thanks in the middle.

Faith thanks God in the middle of the mess,
Faith thanks God in the middle of the night,
Faith thanks God in the middle of the story—
Because it believes in the relentless goodness of
Him who won't stop writing till there's good at the end
of this story.[12]

These words impact me. God is still at work in my story until good comes out of it.

I'm not at the end of my story, at least not yet. I wonder, can good come out of this cancer? This surgery, with all its scars? I can praise God for being good because my faith gives me strength, but for good to come out of my cancer? I wonder, what would that look like? There it is again: a glimmer of curiosity about the good to come.

The Next Part of My Story

I recover quickly after the surgery. Following recommendations for radiation treatment, I wait only three weeks before I begin the anxiety-producing sessions.

Daily, I follow the yellow strip painted along the floor directing patients to the radiation department. The song from *The Wizard of Oz* floats into my mind: "Follow the yellow brick road…" The familiar tune plays over and over in my head, inviting me to join in and sing along. I chuckle to myself. The path I walk may be similar to Dorothy's, although I look down at my runners and lament that my shoes aren't red and fancy like hers.

Dorothy's story takes her along a yellow brick road to find the way home to her family. My goal? Stay healthy as long as I can, so I can spend time with my loved ones.

I consider what it would be like to see a grown, masked woman skip along the yellow line to radiation, singing the popular tune along the way. I imagine people might feel inclined to lead me to another ward, so I instead I just walk normally, although I sing silently the words to the song, humming to fill in the gaps when I forget the lyrics. It helps to distract me from what's coming.

When I get to the treatment room, I look around. It's early and no one is waiting. The place is deserted.

I take a seat across from a row of empty chairs with thick crisscrossed wires tied to their arms. Every second or third chair is adorned with the same big sign that screams:

> 1 OCCUPANT PER BENCH: FOR THE SAFETY OF EVERYONE, PLEASE MAINTAIN ADEQUATE SOCIAL DISTANCE.

The only thing worse than simply having cancer is having cancer during a pandemic when feeling abandoned and alone is the new normal.

The double doors slowly slide open, interrupting my thoughts. A cheerful technician clothed in a long white jacket calls my name. I follow her in, being careful not to touch anything. I quickly strip off my top, my bra, and slide into a hospital gown.

Feeling precariously exposed and insecure, I lie face-up on the cold metallic bed, its slim and sterile frame holding me still. I imagine it tipping over. Two technicians slide a foam wedge under my legs to support my knees and back, then kindly bring me a warm blanket for comfort.

They think of everything.

It takes two of them to gently place the custom-made plastic mesh mask over my still-swollen face and neck. Adorned from the top of my head and extending to my shoulders, I'm concealed behind the mask. They gently pull back my hair so they can tie it into pigtails high above my ears.

First Dorothy, now Pippi Longstocking, I muse. *I wonder who's next?*

They slide my hair through the holes to keep it away from my face. *Snap-snap-snap-snap.* The technicians clip my mask to the table, pinning down my shoulders and head to keep me in place.

Now that I'm secure inside, they slip in the rod-like plastic mouthpiece to keep my jaw open. No moving allowed.

Secured. Pinned in place. Unable to move. I'm afraid to open my eyes in case they get stuck open in the tight mask.

A bubble of claustrophobia slowly rises into my chest. Eyes closed, I try to distract myself.

I practice my relaxation techniques. *Breathe in, breathe out. Count to four, slowly.*

The technicians leave the room and I lie still while they electronically adjust the table from a workstation hidden behind the wall. The adjustments never seem smooth; they're short and abrupt bursts that jiggle the bed into place.

Then, stillness. Silence. I wait.

I think about the loneliness of undergoing surgery and treatment during a pandemic. I sigh and think, *Why do we have to do this alone? It's awfully hard to be doing this alone.* I think about all the research I've read on human attachment and recall that when our hand is held by a loved one, we calm down. Oh, how I wish someone was here to hold my hand.

It starts. The whirring, clicking, and clunking radiation machine calibrates around my head. A beep and then another long *beeeeeepppppp.*

The radiation starts. My anxiety rises in anticipation of the beeping. Anticipation is worse than the treatment itself. I can't feel a thing.

The setup usually takes only minutes—much longer when it's a new technician running the machine. The radiation itself only runs for one to one and a half minutes. I practice holding my breath and not moving. I count, like I did when I was a kid: *Kodak 1, Kodak 2, Kodak 3…* Distraction has become my friend.

Anxiety rises further up my throat. I have to breathe. My brain needs oxygen to calm it down.

In slow 1–2–3–4, out slow 1–2–3–4.

The whole experience causes my heart rate to spike. Intuitively I know it to be truth, even though I can't feel it pounding in my chest. Every muscle is tight and on guard. I only feel anxiety rising in my throat and make a mental note to check my watch later to see how high my heart rate spiked. Days earlier, when I had the mask made in the simulation room, it had risen to over double my regular resting heart rate.

Anxiety too has become a new friend, although it's one I wish would leave me alone.

The technicians whisk in again and praise me for a job well done. They're always here, always cheerful, always kind. These are good people. *Snap-snap-snap-snap.* Once I'm released from the mask, they lift it off just as gently as before.

"You're free now!" one of them says.

They advise me to keep an eye out for the burns along my neck and the mouth sores which are likely to show up. They remind me to apply cream to my neck every day and rinse my mouth regularly.

"And don't worry," they tell me. "If you lose a bit of hair near your neck, it'll probably grow back."

I quickly change back into my top as they sanitize the bed and touchpoints in preparation for the next patient.

As I dress, I glance up at the wall of little box-like compartments, each filled with different types of head masks—some big, others small—for other patients. An empty spot is reserved for mine. My name is neatly typed on the label.

I wonder who these patients are and what their stories entail. It's hard to believe there are so many others like me. My heart swells with compassion. Somehow it gives me solace to remember that I'm not really alone.

I wish I could take a photograph, so I never forget the sight of all those masks. Even without a photo, the image of that wall filled with empty masks and faceless people will stay with me forever.

As I make my way back to the elevator, I pass a mural of a tree painted on the hallway wall. Its leaves are falling off—not down to the ground like normal leaves but floating up and away into the sky. Between the falling leaves, birds are flying free. It's as if the dying leaves have transformed into birds.

Near the tree trunk, I see one single, powerful word: hope. It reminds me that there is always hope available despite the challenges. Like the tree mural, there are seasons of life, death, and second chances with treatment—with an element of rebirth, like the little birds flying free.

A seed of hope is planted in my heart and the warmth of gratitude wells up in me for the gift of a wonderful team of doctors and access to a world-class treatment centre.

I step into the elevator. As it rises, so does my curiosity about how the next part of my story might play out.

Writing Our Stories

It's easy to see our experiences from one perspective—purely negative, and often tied to those unmet expectations about how our story should go. Yet when we can expand that view to welcome other perspectives, we experience life differently.

Many times I don't have the words to express the impact of my experiences. Writing helps me explore my emotions and thoughts. It tends to raise my awareness of what's keeping me stuck. It gives me a chance to ask myself questions aloud I might not consider if I was just thinking silently to myself.

James Pennebaker, an American social psychologist and pioneer in writing therapy, studied the ways in which language and writing can help us deal with emotional upheavals. I have immensely enjoyed his book, *Expressive Writing: Words that Heal*,[13] because of his findings and the practical writing exercises. These exercises help in processing difficult experiences and have helped me gain insights and develop new perspectives by integrating my thoughts and feelings into a coherent story.

Pennebaker's research shows that when we express our highly emotional experiences in words, over time we become less concerned with how they affect us.

His exercises include intentional writing and rewriting about our experiences to help make sense of and process them. In this type of writing, the circumstances don't change, but the writer's understanding and perspectives can. The chief benefit is the ability to release and heal from the memories associated with these experiences, although there are other physical and psychological health benefits. We process our experiences in order to release, to accept, to see new things, to grow, to heal…

I've seen the results firsthand, both with my clients and myself. These exercises helped me decide to write while I was in the hospital, since I knew I wouldn't be able to speak for several days. Throughout the time I was there, I read and journalled daily. During the weeks and months of my recovery, I continued to read and write. I still read and write regularly about my experiences today.

The practice of reflective writing can help us understand, learn, integrate, grow, and heal from our most difficult experiences. Sometimes we can do this alone; other times, we need help from professionals to process the hard stuff.

Transforming Stories

Another author I enjoy reading is Dr. Curt Thompson, MD, a psychiatrist who weaves diverse perspectives together using psychology, neurobiology, and faith to help people cultivate healthy ways of releasing shame and seeing their experiences and stories through a faith-based lens.

In one of Thompson's recent online posts, he wrote that "God is quite intent upon using all of your experiences to draw you into the beauty and goodness that your story is intended to become."[14] And it's all for God's glory, allowing God to be revealed to others through seeing Him at work in us.

I read Thompson's statement out loud. We can be drawn in to see, experience, and show all the beautiful qualities and goodness of God through a cancer journey? How?

As I consider this idea, I try to personalize it. He'll use my experiences to draw me into the beauty and goodness that my story is intended to convey. But is it true that my story is supposed to become beautiful and good? My cancer—with these scars, with this tongue, with a droopy eye? Seriously, how is this possible?

I think back to my experiences in the hospital. Even though there were terribly difficult times, I was able to endure. Sometimes I was even cheerful, celebrating each milestone I reached. I also felt moments of unexplainable hope, peace, and love. Sometimes even some joy. Can this be God's glory? The fruit He bears which comes from His goodness? Is this part of God's goodness—helping me cope and discover hope and understand wholeness differently? Can this taste of wholeness be something that comes from God's spirit too?

But the fruit of the Spirit is love, joy, peace, forbearance,
kindness, goodness, faithfulness, gentleness and self-control.
(Galatians 5:22–23)

Even in the midst of suffering and physical changes, I must embrace new perspectives to come through the other side to experience, accept, and release glimmers of peace, hope, and wholeness.

Opening Up

Back in the hospital, when I had difficulty breathing during the corking procedure, I felt the most vulnerable and alone of any period in my life. I believed that everything had been stripped away from me. But it's also where I learned that God, in the end, is the giver of life and breath. Literally, my breath. And for the first time, in a new way, I realized at a very deep level that God alone is truly enough for me. It was no longer just head knowledge; it was a deep heart knowledge.

Instead of focusing solely on the suffering, our views can expand through cultivating curiosity, openness, and gratitude. As these qualities within us expand, our characters change, our outlook changes, and our relationships change, drawing us into healing and wholeness that can reveal an even greater story than our own.

How we see and interpret these stories has the power to bring new life, growth, and meaning. We can develop the power to impact other people's stories as we celebrate and share with them.

Dan Allender, author of *To Be Told*, writes,

> First, God is not merely the Creator of our life. He is also the Author of our life, and he writes each person's life to reveal his divine story. There never has been nor ever will be another life like mine—or like yours. Just as there is only one face and name like mine, so there is only one story like mine. And God writes the story of my life to make something known about himself, the One who wrote me. The same is true of you. Your

life and mine not only reveal who we are, but they also help reveal who God is.[15]

If God is a good God, and if He created us to bear His image, and if He defines our identity as one of value, and if He has authored our story from past to present, and if He is the one who will continue writing into the future, then we can trust that there is a good purpose and meaning in the story we are currently living.

We need to look backwards, look at the present moment, and look into the future to see and better understand God's full story as our own.

As I've already mentioned, crises have a way of shaking what we once thought we knew—our understanding, identity, values, and belief systems. Crises also present a unique opportunity for us to examine and update what we believe and trust, giving us the ability to participate in the writing of a new chapter of our unfolding story.

When our faith and trust wanes, circumstances can begin to overwhelm us. Trusting that God is a good God, and that His promises are true, brings us hope. Even when our circumstances are difficult, by holding on to faith and trust in God's goodness we can see more clearly, enabling us to regain strength and hope.

In many cases, we can't change the past or our circumstances. But we can influence how we see them and uncover helpful ways to process their impact. As we do this, we can find new purpose and meaning instead of letting circumstances dictate them, lest they turn us into victims.

We aren't victims of our stories.

We are sojourners, and along the way some challenges we face will be horribly difficult. Other experiences will be delightful. They can be both good and bad at the same time.

Yet our circumstances only tell part of the story. When we become curious about God's bigger story and learn what it is, our perspective changes. This can influence how our future unfolds.

Cultivating Curiosity

When I remember to cultivate curiosity about my own circumstances and ask questions that challenge my thinking, I see things differently.

I become more open to welcoming mystery instead of thinking in dualistic ways. In this manner, I become better able to make helpful decisions and live in ways that bring greater wholeness.

The adventure I'm currently on presents me with the opportunity to embrace the life I have and live it as well as I can along the road of recovery with all its sorrow, pain, and limitation. At the same time, I can embrace wonderful new experiences that bring me hope and lead to building new relationships that teach me what's truly important in life. This is a time when I can come to deeply understand the source of my hope and redefine my understanding of wholeness.

In any crisis or challenge, I try to ask myself a series of practical questions to help cultivate curiosity:

- Where does my mind spend most of its time—in the present, past, or future? Or do I spend my time fantasizing? If it's the future, what am I worried about? If it's the past, what am I regretting? If it's the present, what challenge am I facing? If I'm fantasizing or daydreaming, what do I really want or need?
- How much of my time is spent dwelling on the crisis? What are my feelings relating to this? Name them.
- What other perspectives can I use to look at this situation? How do these other perspectives make me feel? Give each a name.
- If I were to give myself a time limit each day to focus on this issue, what other things could fill my thoughts or my day that would bring joy?
- What specific things was I grateful for before this crisis that I still have? What did that gratitude feel like? Try to experience that feeling now. Am I still grateful for those things? Write them down and keep a daily record.
- Who are the people in my life—family, friends, other supports, etc.—for whom I can be grateful today?
- What are my expectations? My desires?

- What do I have control over? What don't I have control over?
- What expectations or desires do I hold onto that make me feel like a victim or prevent me from healing and feeling whole? Do I need to spend some time grieving these losses?
- What parts of this journey still bring me angst, excessive worry, or other unhelpful behaviour?
- What kinds of new perspectives, decisions, goals, or plans can I make to help me work through these unhelpful issues?
- What do I want to see happen? What do I need? Who can help me? What resources are available to me?
- How can I extend some self-compassion to myself?
- What is one simple thing I can do that brings me joy, pleasure, or a sense of peace?
- What do I need to remember that is good, true, and filled with hope?
- In this journey I'm on, what kind of person do I want to be?

Writing out the answers, without succumbing to the urge to vent, helps me process what I'm going through. What I find interesting is that when I write it all down, I feel better—sometimes right away, sometimes the next day. And if it's too much to do alone, I ask for some quality time with someone who can help me process.

Or I'll try the Pennebaker approach once I understand what's holding me back. It's as though I'm emptying out all the stuff rolling around in my head. When I empty out the clutter, I seem to have more room to understand my experiences and emotions, and in the end this helps me figure out what I need to do next.

Sometimes I keep what I write. Other times I shred it. The shredding, in many ways, is cathartic because it symbolizes a release or letting go of what can no longer be. Then I can let a new chapter begin, figuratively speaking.

Things to Remember

Along the way toward healing and wholeness, I find it helps to give myself clear reminders of those things in which I've always had faith and trust:

- Knowing and regularly reminding myself of the promises found in Romans 8:28 helps me to continue looking forward with expectancy to how God will use the experience I'm going through right now.
- I can acknowledge and lament the pain and suffering in my life without losing hope. I can suffer well and even suffer with joy without minimizing or denying the accompanying pain or challenges.
- I can acknowledge that there is no hierarchy of suffering—even when others compare their illnesses or losses to mine. No one's crisis is greater or lesser than another's. All suffering is difficult. And we all suffer. Comparison only brings shame. It pushes out empathy, love, and compassion, creating isolation and disconnection.

Being curious helps me to discover new viewpoints and courage. When I try seeing things from different perspectives, I can gain new insights.

When I need comfort, I can remind myself that God never leaves us alone. It's when I feel alone that my focus slips from hope to discouragement. When I see myself as a victim, I can't see beyond that victim label. Yet when I see myself as a person of value, one who is designed to heal and be whole while being filled with hope of a good future, whether here on earth or in heaven, I can thrive.

God's invitation to me is something I can accept with faith and trust, or reject and choose something else. Every time I have accepted this invitation, I have grown, healed, and felt more whole. Best of all, I have become a more authentic version of myself. This can only have a positive impact on others in my circles too.

And every time I have rejected this offer, I've gotten stuck, forgotten where I find my hope, and suffered more. This too impacts others.

One way has an impact that brings life; the other way doesn't.

Believing that God promises to bring good out of difficult situations helps me cultivate a greater level of gratitude for the challenges in my life. This is the truth I choose to believe, even if I don't yet see the end of the story. Trusting God brings me hope. It also sows seeds of hope which produce much gratitude, even in the middle of the story when the ending is unknown.

Cultivating gratitude about God's ability to redeem any situation is a way to live deeply in our faith. Remembering that God is good, that He wants good for us, and that He can work in every circumstance for good helps us to keep working toward wholeness with hope.

> *And we know that in all things God works for the good of those who love him, who have been called according to his purpose.* (Romans 8:28)

And while we keep remembering, moving from moment to moment, we develop a deeper reliance on God, especially in our weakness, by praying for strength, hope, wisdom, and insight. We learn to trust in His promise to redeem all things so that eventually we will be made fully whole again.

HIGHLIGHTS

We were designed by God to be whole. That's a part of His story for us. It's a part of our story too. This was the original plan for mankind.

Reflections
Consider What Keeps Us Stuck

- Becoming whole doesn't mean getting fixed or going back to life as it was. That's impossible because every crisis changes us.
- Our stories may be difficult, but we aren't victims of our stories.

Consider What Brings Life

- If God is good, and if He created us to bear His image, and if He defines our identity as one of value, and if He has authored our story from past to present, and if He is the one who will continue writing into the future, then we can trust that there is good purpose and meaning in the story we are currently living.
- Our story isn't over yet because God isn't done until good comes from it.
- In many cases, we can't change the past or our circumstances.
- But we can influence how we see those circumstances and uncover helpful ways to process their impact.
- Cultivating gratitude about God's ability to redeem any situation is a way to live deeply in our faith. Remembering that God is good, that He wants good for us, and that He can work in every circumstance for good helps us keep working toward wholeness with hope.

Personal Reflection

- What is your usual or favoured way to process experiences you are trying to make sense of? What is one thing you can do to begin developing a new means of processing your experiences that might bring you new insight or hope?

- Have you ever considered where your mind spends most of its time? In the past, present, future, or fantasizing? Reflect on what this means to you.

- What is one manageable topic you can use to practice using some of the questions listed in this chapter to reflect on and journal about?

Chapter Four

PERSEVERANCE

"Well," said the King at last, "we must go on and
take the adventure that comes to us."[16]
—C.S. Lewis

A JOURNEY TAKES US places. Sometimes the journey is easy whereas other
times it's challenging, leading us to depths or heights we never imagined.
The way in which we interpret our challenges impacts our future
decisions, the direction we take, and our ability to cope and persevere
through it all.

Acknowledging when a problem exists can help us determine what
resources are best needed to help us. When we choose helpful resources,
we tend to be more optimistic, cope better, and persevere. As a result,
our resiliency grows. And as we become more resilient, we become better
equipped to persevere.

If at First You Don't Succeed
I learned this firsthand on a trip to Spain a few years ago. One of the
best privileges extended to me during my retirement has been to travel
overseas offering workshops to teams of international workers.

On the first trip to Spain, I finish my workshop a bit early and leave
our friends, who are the team leaders, to conduct individual meetings
with their staff. We decide to take advantage of the daylight to go
sightseeing.

Spain is beautiful, especially in the small towns near Madrid. One
town we visit is full of medieval history and culture. At every corner,

historic buildings loom overhead, each with huge bird nests belonging to long-legged white storks. Religious buildings stand on every other corner, home to the diverse Jewish, Muslim, and Christian communities who live in harmony there.

My husband downloads a simple tourist map before we venture out. Map in hand, we confidently begin our adventure. We walk briskly in the crisp air, searching for the main entrance as we near the walled city. We stop frequently to snap photos of the beautiful buildings.

The main entrance is nowhere to be found. We assume we missed it and decide to keep walking, only to stumble upon a small side entrance. In we go with renewed energy, ready and excited to explore the city centre.

Lights shine from overhead along the narrow cobblestone streets. Vendor kiosks line the square, their shopkeepers standing shoulder to shoulder while music blares from speakers positioned high on poles. As the evening arrives, the crowd grows to fill the square and join the festivities. It's Christmas time and the market square buzzes.

Two hours pass, and we realize that darkness is quickly settling in. It's time to head back to eat, rest, and review our sessions for the next day and wait for our friends to return from their meetings.

We look left, then right. Which way do we go?

With greater scrutiny, we realize that the map doesn't show every road. It only shows the most popular parts of the inner city and we can't figure out how to return.

My heart sinks.

We decide to look for the main entrance by walking along the road adjacent to the fortress wall. Sooner or later, we figure we'll find the entrance.

But after ten minutes, we realize we are hopelessly lost.

This is the second time I've become lost in a foreign country where I don't speak the language. The first time, I was in a car by myself in Poland, trying to find a friend's house outside of Warsaw. The difference between now and then? When I was alone, there was no one to disagree with about directions.

I don't read or speak Spanish. I'm strong in French, but not Spanish. Even though the two languages have significant similarities, they're still different languages. I can figure out some words, but it's still challenging. Therefore, some signage we pass goes undeciphered.

We try our best to remember the twists and turns taken earlier, but we pass several roadways, detours, and buildings. They're too numerous to count and it's impossible to figure out where we are. My legs throb with each step we take along the uneven roadway.

Sighing, we try to backtrack and consult with each other at every corner, wondering, "Does this look familiar?"

Finally, my husband decides we should go one way and I believe it's the other way. However, I have this rule while on holidays: I don't like getting annoyed or getting into arguments. It can ruin an otherwise good memory.

Therefore, with every ounce of self-control I can muster, I bite my tongue and agree to try his way—first. After all, I remind myself, he has a pretty good ability to find his way around back home. Often better than me. But he never, ever asks for help if he does become lost.

A knot forms in my stomach and moves up into my chest as the frustration rises. I hate wasting time and, in my opinion, getting lost qualifies as a huge waste of time. I tend to be proactive and forecast upcoming issues to mitigate their negative impacts; my husband tends to be reactive, going with the flow and figuring out how to solve a problem as it evolves. Usually we balance each other out quite well, but in times when our personality differences clash I catch myself wondering how we can possibly be so different.

They say opposites attract! Most times everything works out, but not when we're lost in a country where we can't speak the language.

I've learned that some people don't willingly ask for help. They just keep exploring until they find their way—eventually. No matter how long it takes. My husband is one of those types. He is in absolutely no rush, ever.

We realize that we don't even know the address to our apartment, though, so we can't ask for directions. We just know it by sight. If we get close enough, we'll recognize the neighbourhood, stores, and street.

We walk for twenty minutes, passing corner after corner, the streetlights aglow as they illumine our way in the dusk. Nothing appears familiar. We plod past many a restaurant, the most delicious aromas wafting through the air. Hunger and exhaustion feed my growing annoyance.

With no margin left, I do the only thing I can do—I start to complain about my sore legs and back. At every second block, I'm compelled to sit down and rest.

After taking a few deep breaths, I remember that we'd been taking photos all day and wonder if we can use those photos to retrace our steps. Excited about the possibility, we sit shoulder to shoulder, our heads together bent over the tablet. We scroll through the photos.

Hope renewed, we head back until we find a place we both recognize from our photos.

We take another moment to our rest our sore legs and scour the photos again until we see the landmark matching the building in front of us. These landmarks keep pointing us in the direction we need to go, and painstakingly we find our way out the side gate we entered through just hours earlier.

With relief, we slowly trudge along the main road heading toward our apartment.

Along the way, we catch sight of a huge gate. We look at each other in amazement, then summon the courage to peek through to see what's inside. We recognize some of the buildings we photographed and realize we had been only moments from the exit all along. Our sense of humour returns, and we laugh at our predicament, wondering how we could have missed it.

We grab groceries at the local store, then return home and eat supper. Thoroughly exhausted, we head to bed. My husband decides to leave the key in the double-bolted lock to make it easier to let in our friends when they get back later, saving us from having to fumble around for the keys in the dark.

About an hour into our exhausted slumber, our friends return to the apartment. *Knock-knock-knock. Ring-ring-ring.* Nothing rouses us. We are deeply asleep.

Disappointed, our equally exhausted friends walk back to the train terminal and climb aboard to return to their colleagues' house to spend the night.

Waking up the next morning, I think to myself, *Wow, those guys are super quiet. I didn't hear them come in last night.*

I slip out of bed, tiptoe around the corner, and peek into their room—only to find their bedroom door wide open, the bed neatly made.

Unknown to us, the European-built door has a safety feature that stops any other key from opening it from the outside when keys are inserted from the inside. Even with good intentions, what we knew would have worked at home didn't work here, in a different context. Little could we have known that something we'd done to make things easier would turn out to be such a hindrance.

Although this is a somewhat funny story, we can learn from it.

The resources we use in coping with a crisis don't come with a guarantee that our expected outcomes will occur. There are always other external influences. In not recognizing the assumptions we make and not testing our resources in different contexts, our chosen tools can make a situation worse, causing stress and inconvenience and even affecting our ability to persevere.

We need to develop and access tools like knowing the values that drive our behaviour, cultivating curiosity about challenges we face, and choosing to embrace hope-filled optimism. These will make us more resilient when difficult times strike—and as we build that resilience, we will be better able to persevere.

Knowing Our Values

Sometimes knowing our values can be a useful guide during a crisis, helping us to persevere and better understand our motivations.

While visiting Spain, we valued rest, full tummies, and safety, as well as being professionally prepared for our session the next day. That's what motivated us to keep trying to find a way to get home.

Values are the things we believe are of greatest importance in how we live our lives. They typically focus on the present moment and can serve as a standard from which we make choices and use resources.

For example, if we truly value our health and well-being, we'll make choices to care for the physical, emotional, spiritual, and social parts of ourselves. We might intentionally maintain an active lifestyle, exercise regularly, eat well, get our rest, grow spiritually, and stay connected in healthy community. This doesn't mean we have to be perfect all the time, but it means that overall we take care of ourselves on an ongoing basis in the best way we are able. And on days when we forget, or choose not to take these actions, we can learn from our behaviour.

Living from our values isn't just a desire or wish; it's about a deep-seated need that motivates us—that is, if we don't ignore our values, suppress them, or allow our emotions to overtake us and cause us to react automatically. It's about cultivating greater awareness so we can persevere on an ongoing basis.

Persevere means "continue steadfastly, persist."[17] What stands out most to me in that definition is the word continue and its Latin roots: "join together in uninterrupted succession, make or be continuous, do successively one after another…"[18]

These words, taken together, make me consider whether perseverance is experienced as a succession of efforts that align with our values, instead of a one-and-done exercise. Such intentional efforts may require us to re-evaluate or adjust our use of a resource that might not have worked in a specific context. In such a moment, if one effort fails we can learn from it and try something else. It's all part of persevering.

When we try to persevere, but end up slipping and failing, we aren't failures but learners.

When we try to persevere, but end up slipping and failing, we aren't failures but learners. We're on our way, learning to persevere because of what we value. And as we continue to make decisions based on our values, we embrace a more congruent, unfragmented way of life.

When our thoughts and behaviours line up with our values—when what we think, say, and do matches what we believe and value—it fuels our ability to persevere. Our style of values-based perseverance becomes an additional resource for us to use in our pursuit of wholeness.

Hope-Filled Optimism

We all respond differently to a crisis. Our thoughts, emotions, and responses impact our ability to persevere. Some suggest that we need to be more positive; others say that being positive can be toxic. Some suggest that venting helps; others say that too much negativity can be toxic too.

With toxic positivity, a person's words could be taken as being dismissive of a difficult situation by being overly cheerful about a crisis. Basically, it's possible to minimize a challenge by ignoring, suppressing, or denying the reality of one's emotions.

With toxic negativity, a person exaggerates a difficult situation by focusing only on the negative and discounting any good.

Toxic positivity and toxic negativity are extremes. Both are unhelpful in terms of developing perseverance.

For myself, I've chosen hope-filled optimism—a type of optimism that acknowledges a person's difficult emotions and the challenges brought on by a crisis. But that isn't all. It's also hopeful in its ability to see opportunities amidst those challenges, allowing the difficult experiences to change us. Hope-filled optimism helps us see the reality of a difficult situation, cope in helpful ways, gain new insight, and make meaning from the experience. It's about believing unrelentingly that our crises will be redeemed and that the future holds hope, both here on earth and in heaven.

Hope-filled optimism helps cultivate perseverance because it possesses a growth mindset that acknowledges difficulties, admitting that there is much we don't understand, while also looking for what is good. Good in the circumstances. Good in people. It looks for what is hopeful. It looks for the opportunities in an experience, while also accepting that there may be times when waves of grief and emotions surface.

> **Hope-filled optimism helps cultivate perseverance because it possesses a growth mindset...**

There are times, early in a crisis, when we need extra support and compassion. But over time, if we process and integrate our experiences, we will change, grow, and heal.

The need for support and compassion usually diminishes. As we heal and become stronger, we become better able to cope and reintegrate into daily life. We can use our crisis experience to serve and support others who are going through their own difficult times. And in so doing, we can bear witness to the gift of perseverance and hope amidst suffering.

Holding steadfast with patience and cultivating optimism that brings with it hope and perseverance allows us to endure through a crisis. This combination of steadfastness and hopeful optimism helps us discover alternative solutions, helps us cope, and helps us manoeuvre through crises while acknowledging that we can find silver linings.

When we find a middle ground between toxic extremes, we can gain new perspectives by not discounting the positive or negative impacts of our situation. This will guide us into finding new resources and building resilience to persevere through our present situation and cultivate a mindset of optimism.

Resilience skills, like hope-filled optimism, can help us accept suffering and find ways to see opportunities for change. These skills help us clear from our minds the unhelpful clutter.

Cultivating Curiosity

Cultivating resilience often allows for us gain new insights into the reality of our limitations, giving us a clearer view of what our needs are while compassionately acknowledging challenges. Resilience also helps us to remember what's good in life without dismissing the parts that bring good change. Resiliency helps us persevere because we're able to bounce back.

If we can look at our circumstances with a heart of curiosity, another resilience skill, instead of judgment—by giving things labels for being good or bad—it will fan faith, trust, and hope within us. This type of mindset can even bring with it an anticipation of what is to come. It doesn't deny the emotions or challenges experienced, but it does open our minds and hearts to see what's right before us in the here and now.

Holding this perspective can also expand our view to include the good happening around us, allowing us to draw strength from it. This helps us to become grateful for the simple things in life and take fewer things for granted.

Curiosity and optimism help break our overly positive or negative tendencies and make room for more helpful thinking that brings in hope, wholeness, and redemptive healing. When this happens, we can come to see ourselves, others, and even God differently, more accurately, and with more awareness and gratitude. We can see the crisis from a wider vantage point by stepping back and being curious, acknowledging challenges while also reminding ourselves about the things for which we are grateful.

It is important to attend to the questions, concerns, and emotions that arise in this process, because they can be life-changing. We have the choice to receive, dismiss, or ignore these opportunities.

When received, they can impact our development and cause us to grow and uncover new ways in which we can relate to one another and to God. These opportunities often help us mature and become less fragmented, able to see others and the world with curiosity; we become more tender, compassionate, authentic, forgiving, and loving.

This is the kind of wonderful opportunity we are presented with in a crisis. We can grow and change for the better through it instead of getting bitter or resentful.

Resilience skills like optimism and curiosity bring about opportunities to embrace peace, strength, compassion, and hope while building perseverance in us. Even when things may be challenging, when we pay attention to what's around us and notice the good, no matter how small, we tend to see greater amounts of good and find more for which to be grateful.

A Few Observations

As I enter my retirement years, I have more time to show how greatly I value my relationships with God, my husband, my children, my grandchildren, my extended family, and my friends. My retirement plans originally included being the best grandparent ever, to have some fun traveling with my husband while also painting, writing, and volunteering to give back to my community.

Then the pandemic hit, and immediately after—cancer. Within months, my family and friends were struck with multiple health crises, eight of them within a ten-month period. All my retirement plans came to a screeching halt.

Never once had any of my plans taken into account a pandemic, nor a threatening health crisis for myself, my husband, or our unborn granddaughter. And they certainly didn't account for the death or illness of dear friends within the same year as my diagnosis.

These crises have forced me to find new resources, or hone old ones, so I could learn, grow, and cultivate curiosity and a mindset of daily coping and perseverance. Knowing who and what I value has helped me set priorities and make decisions that keep me persevering and cultivating a hopeful attitude.

Now here I am in the latter part of my life, a cancer survivor who's immunocompromised by medication that I need to take to keep an autoimmune disease in remission. I'm also living a somewhat healthy, relatively active, simple yet full lifestyle that brings me joy, gratitude, and hope every day.

My plans haven't materialized the way I dreamed they would. Many surprises and disappointments have required me to make difficult decisions and take unexpected directions. And although the pain, loss, and suffering I've experienced most recently are the most difficult I have had to contend with, I am extremely grateful for how I've grown and for what I've learned. I have a lot for which to be thankful. I am grateful for many special faithful people in my life. Cultivating a mindset of curiosity, optimism, and knowing my values has a played key role in developing the ability to persevere and find hope.

I have some amazing new people in my life. I've built deeper and more intimate relationships with some of my long-term friends. I am continually inspired by others who go through life demonstrating perseverance and hope.

My husband and I are also closer and appreciate each other in new ways. We laugh more and appreciate the little things we once took for granted. I cherish the time we spend with our children and grandchildren more than ever because I'm unsure what the future holds.

At every turn, I want to let others know that I appreciate them and am grateful for who they are. I try to focus on that which brings goodness and lightness to my heart while trying to cherish every moment without denying the challenges that may arise. I want to embrace joy and see fruit through my interactions with others, trying not to take anything for granted. I want to be grateful for them all, because each person in my life is a special gift.

When I know what I value in life, I can analyze the choices I make to see if they draw me closer to living out my values or further away. Am I growing closer to God, or away from God? Closer to people, or away from people? Closer to peace, joy, and hope, or away from it?

I have changed and grown because of my cancer experience. I'm freer to be me, limitations and all. Best of all, I'm filled with renewed hope in every part of my life—in my relationships, in my faith, in my health, in my activities, and in my future.

Optimism cultivates perseverance, and perseverance cultivates strength of character in us to find hope. When we find hope, we become more resilient. As we become more resilient, we often find joy because of where we place our hope.

I wish I hadn't needed to go through some of these severe experiences to learn and grow in this way, but I am beyond grateful for the outcomes—the personal, emotional, and spiritual growth. I'm different now than I was before. I'm still me, but I think and hope I am a better version of me.

Yet without these recent challenges, I would not have had the opportunity to grow, change, and learn the gifts of perseverance and strength because of the hope I have embraced.

My strategies for coping served me well in the past, but each one needed to be updated for my specific challenges; they needed to be aligned with what I value. Just like the story about accidentally locking our friends out of our apartment, the old ways that had worked in the past can accidentally work against the good. The map we had thought would be a helpful tool in reaching our goal did not function in the way we assumed.

The Benefit of Perseverance

The effort expended in persevering is often challenging. But the effort is worthwhile because we become more resilient in the process. How we persevere is affected by our values, beliefs, outlook, expectations, and automatic reactions when things go wrong.

We don't realize how distracting our expectations and assumptions are until a crisis hits, squeezing out the hidden things deep in our hearts. When they're finally exposed, they make us question our identity, values, past, and future—pretty much everything we once believed to be true.

Crises have a way of turning our world on its head, messing up our plans and dreams. They make us rethink what we believe and what we expect from life. They even have a dangerous way of distracting us and making us forget who we really are, forcing us to give up parts of who we are and how we have been designed to be—whole.

Reacting to a crisis without considering how our thoughts, expectations, or assumptions impact us will affect our ability to persevere, often negatively.

The crisis itself can bring gifts of opportunity to see ourselves, others, and the world more clearly, to identify what we truly value, and to find ways to live from these values. These are opportunities to choose to live well amidst suffering and embrace it. We can live well despite not knowing our futures.

We all face struggles.

We all suffer.

We all grieve.

Eventually, we all die.

And we all have a choice about how to find a way to live well along the way through knowing our values, being curious, embracing optimism, persevering, and finding hope that brings life and wholeness.

A blessing awaits us as we persevere and look for these answers that bring life and wholeness. They were hidden before. They are unfolding now. They will be revealed in full later.

As we grow in our ability to persevere, we will uncover glimpses of the next chapter in our story, which produces even more hope for us.

HIGHLIGHTS

A blessing awaits us as we persevere, looking for these answers that bring life and wholeness. They were hidden before. They are unfolding now. They will be revealed in full later.

Reflections

Consider What Keeps Us Stuck

- Toxic positivity and toxic negativity are extremes. Both are unhelpful in terms of developing perseverance.

Consider What Brings Life

- Knowing our values during a crisis can sometimes be useful in terms of choosing a helpful resource.
- Hope-filled optimism helps cultivate perseverance because it produces a growth mindset that acknowledges difficulties while also looking for what's good.
- Days of crisis can produce opportunities for us to choose to live well amidst suffering to persevere and find hope.

Personal Reflection

- Think of a situation you recently experienced. Where did you place most of your focus? How much of your focus was placed on the negatives versus the positives? Reflect on the impact each thinking style had on you.
- What is one thing you are optimistic about today? Think about things in the past you were grateful for: a fresh cup of coffee, tea with a friend, a walk in a park, warm sun on your face, a word of kindness, a smile, waking up in a warm, cozy bed, etc.
- Think of things you have experienced in the present that recently that brought pleasure: singing a song, reading an encouraging quote or good book, taking a

call from a friend, etc. What is one thing you can do more of this week?

• Throughout the day, look for one thing that brings you feelings of peace, joy, hopefulness, goodness, connection, contentment, or pleasure for any of your senses—sight, sound, taste, smell, and touch.

Chapter Five

GRIEF AND MOURNING

You never know how much you really believe
anything until its truth or falsehood becomes a
matter of life and death to you.[19]

—C.S. Lewis

WHEN TRAGEDY STRIKES, I usually want to run away by pretending like it never happened. Sometimes I try soothing myself by fantasizing that I can change things—but it's never long before I realize this way of thinking isn't helpful.

I cannot change the past. It's better if I do the hard work of acceptance and healing. Somehow I need to find a way to accept and deal with what I'm facing while keeping in mind that I'm still in the middle of my life's story.

When crises hit, I always look for answers. And, if I'm being honest, maybe I want to find a reason to assign blame. Then maybe I could become angry about all the changes I face.

Instead it just makes me sad. I still have no clue *why* I ended up with cancer. I can't become angry at anyone or blame anything or anyone— not even myself. On one hand, I don't have the lifestyle risks; on the other, I still don't know what to discontinue to prevent further risk. This dilemma keeps me stuck in fear.

As if any of it's under my control.

Now I live in a place of ambiguity. I call it the place of not knowing. A place where I have no other option but to trust. Trust God. Trust my doctors. Trust myself too, to make wise choices. The story isn't over until good has come out of it.

Intuitively I recognize that I'm struggling for control—control of my health, control of my life—because in the beginning everything seemed so out of control.

After experiencing a trauma, medical or otherwise, most of us need to regain a sense of control to recover our equilibrium. I am no different. I frequently struggle with the thought that if I knew what to stop doing to reduce my chances of a recurrence of cancer, it would be much easier to prepare and cope. Then I could fix things.

But the reality is that I can fix absolutely nothing about my condition. I must live with an unsettling degree of mystery and chance. Yet it leads me to find good by seeking and savouring joy in each day, each moment, and hang on to hope. It helps me to live more fully in the present and appreciate what I do have and be grateful for those around me.

Each month, I become more adept at learning how to live well with hope while facing an unknown future, no matter the outcome. It's an ongoing process wherein I must release that which holds me back from healing—like my need to have my normal life back, to know the whys, or to control my surroundings.

I'm learning to trust with a degree of emotional vulnerability which is extremely uncomfortable for me. It involves deep levels of trust. Trust in God. Trust in others. Trust in my doctors. Trust in myself and my own ability to choose well.

Trust every single day.

Trusting God is important. I trust God for the outcome, whichever way it goes. I trust in God's goodness and His promises. God cares for us and wants what is best for us.

Trusting my doctors is important too. I trust them to care for me as best they can, because it's why they do what they do, and I know without a doubt that they want good outcomes for me as well.

Trusting myself involves listening to my thoughts and knowing what I tend to avoid or react to so I can make informed choices to better care for myself and my soul.

If I choose to, I could easily feed my continual longing for the unfulfilled dreams I can never have. This would keep me stuck because it wouldn't help me accept the reality of the permanency of my losses. Becoming stuck can lead anyone to discouragement and a victim mindset.

Instead I have developed a habit of looking for the good, the beauty, and the opportunity—especially with broken things. Because when I intentionally look for good, I see more good.

When I look with hope, without dismissing the difficult moments, I see good in people, good in things, good in circumstances, and good in outcomes. Doing this brings me more hope, reminding me of all my blessings. Holding this perspective helps me appreciate the simple joys in life each day and gives me courage to release the false hope of living my old normal.

Deep down I know that this desire to return to my old normal can never to be fulfilled. A return to that way of life is impossible. Only a new normal lies ahead, and I fully trust that God will continue to bring good from it. That is my new hope.

Processing Grief with Art

It's Friday morning. I lounge at the art desk we temporarily moved into our bright, cozy family room. I sip hot coffee and gaze out through the double French doors, admiring the beauty of the white, snow-covered trees.

I have enrolled in an online watercolour class for cancer patients, led by an art therapist. I joined the class partly out of curiosity and partly out of my need for connection, ongoing support, and healing with other cancer patients. No one in this group knows me, so I can hide my profession, and the online format makes it safe to connect while maintaining enough distance to protect myself from having to be vulnerable.

The session is structured with activities and includes watercolour painting, reflective meditation, and sharing. Today the facilitator introduces the art of kintsugi. She explains the artistic style of restoration something like this.

Imagine owning a beautiful bowl, one you cherish. Maybe it has been a family heirloom passed down through the generations. Somehow, it accidentally breaks. Many of us would be heartbroken and attempt to repair it. But we may only be able to see it as damaged goods and either hide it in the back of a cabinet or throw it away.

In the Japanese art of kintsugi, the broken bowl isn't swept aside, nor is it discarded. It is kept solely because it's cherished—even when damaged. An artist is called in to restore it. With kintsugi, the artist's gentle, loving hands can see beauty in its brokenness. With this vision in mind, the confident artist sets about to recover its beauty. The broken bowl is gently yet painstakingly glued back together. Its ragged cracks are then carefully adorned with gold. The artist skillfully paints gold over every broken part to restore it and make it whole—rendering it even more valuable in its brokenness.

Tenderly restored. Made whole. Made new. Made more valuable than before.

Such a restoration process is founded in compassion and patience led by great insight into the beauty of the creator's original handiwork.

In pencil, I lightly sketch out several small bowls, all different sizes and shapes. Then I add jagged lines representing the broken pieces glued back together. I paint each bowl a different colour. Then, with a thin brush, I carefully outline each crack with gold paint to remind me that the bowls are even more beautiful and valuable after they go through the process of restoration.

It's early in my recovery. With a long sigh, I recognize my deep longing to be saved from the trajectory I'm on, yet I sadly acknowledge that healing can only come by going through it. I must be patient with the process and do the work to heal.

I always encouraged my clients to trust the process, so I quietly remind myself, *"Trust the healing process. It takes time. This time is necessary."*

I replay the concepts behind the beautiful process of kintsugi and mindfully continue painting to refocus my mind and heart on the hope that comes through the process of restoration. Bit by bit, a crack seems to heal deep down inside my heart. Restoration is a slow process. It's not my timing that counts. It's the Restorer's job to set the timing for healing.

I remind myself that God is where I find my hope; He is the ultimate restorer of broken hearts. Like the kintsugi artist, He restores with compassion, patience, and love. He already knows our value and beauty. Bit by bit, He restores our hearts in ways that affirm our value and beauty—because He already sees all of us. He brings special people into our lives who can sojourn with us as we heal.

I wonder, when we embrace our brokenness and imperfections, can we too begin to see more clearly how our own brokenness restored can become more beautiful and valuable than it was in its original form?

I trace the edge of the soft scar tissue of the donor site on my arm. I run my finger along the length of the two-and-a-half- by three-inch patch on the wrist, then move up along the long scar that curves up to meet the inside of my elbow where the nerve was removed. Gently, I follow the scar on my neck behind my ear, slowly following it down to the front of my throat and then over my tracheostomy scar.

All scars. All necessary for healing.

Maybe these scars are like the lines of painted gold, part of the restoration process, taken with gentle, meticulous care by my team of skilled surgeons. They are visible reminders of the cancer that's been removed. The scars are like gold, reminding me of what was needed to be taken away to remove the cancer.

Instead of seeing myself as damaged goods or my scars as unsightly, the marks can remind me of my value and of the painstaking care my surgeons took in restoring me back to health.

I choose to let the scars speak of my path of restoration toward wholeness and health. I decide not to hide my scars anymore, but to wear them proudly as a reminder of the miracle of all who were involved in saving my life with such skill, precision, patience, and care because of their dedication and love for humankind.

Strokes of Gold

The inches of visible scars, not to mention the tongue flap which swells regularly and produces a speech impediment that makes me self-conscious, causes my cancer experience to be very public.

At first I was embarrassed to speak because I form words more slowly. I chose clothes carefully with the intention of hiding my scars and avoided speaking to avoid invasive questions from complete strangers. Having cancer, I've learned, is a little like being pregnant. For some curious reason, I become a public curiosity; many feel free to verbalize opinions about my scars, or condition, and often feel compelled to tell comparable horror stories about themselves or others.

But after a while I realized that this must be an automatic reaction to a trigger when people are faced with a hard to imagine type of human suffering. They desperately search for ways to connect to my story without really knowing how. Yet in their discomfort, their words fail to create empathy. I have learned that I can encourage them in their struggle without seeking empathy from them.

My scars and physical changes are a part of the new me and I need to accept me as I am. They don't define who I am; they just represent a difficult experience I've been through. I don't want to be known only as a cancer patient.

I can hide all my other health conditions well, but not this one. It's on display daily. It's easily seen and heard. At first, it challenged my beliefs about what is feminine, attractive, or comfortable for others to be around—until I learned about the act of skilled kintsugi restoration.

It's Okay to Ask

About six months after my surgery, my husband and I host a backyard breakfast with some friends visiting from overseas. Just as they're about to leave, the husband, a former colleague of mine who also possesses a hilarious and somewhat outspoken sense of humour, asks a question that hasn't ever been asked.

After hearing how my tongue was reconstructed, he can't contain his curiosity any longer: "So what's it like to kiss your wife now?"

A little taken aback, and thoroughly embarrassed at the unexpected question, I shyly lean forward to hear my husband's answer.

A loud, deafening silence ensues. All eyes are on my husband as he shifts his weight from one foot to the other.

"Oh! I'd say… it's very good…" He pauses for effect and grins widely. "I'd say it's just like normal."

With that, everyone bursts out laughing. The cancer ice has been broken.

After our friends leave, even though I've asked before, I question my husband about what it's *really* like to kiss me.

"Just like normal," he repeats, pulling me close. "I can't really tell the difference. Anyway, it's all still part of you."

I snuggle my face deeply into the crook of his neck, my grateful tears falling quietly onto his shirt. Knowing that my husband of forty-three years still finds me attractive, despite all the scars and alterations, is deeply healing.

I welcome another stroke of gold over the cracks, taking one step closer to accepting the new me.

Something that was broken but truly restored is indeed more beautiful and valuable than it was in its original form. Kind, loving words from safe people like my husband can help in the restoration and healing process.

The gold for me is found through my interactions and relationships—God first, then my husband, my family, my friends, and my doctors. Each member of my community, with their faithful, loving care and encouragement, is a kintsugi artist. Each uniquely plays a part in my ongoing restoration. I am extremely grateful for each one of them. They leave behind a little bit of gold in my heart, helping me to heal, become whole, and feel valued and cherished.

Loss and Suffering

Losses challenge us in many ways, bringing pain, suffering, and sorrow. It isn't uncommon to resent losses when they enter our lives. They can challenge our thoughts and belief systems, everything we once knew to be true.

When losses happen, we often label all the emotions we have as grief, because we don't have a name for the myriad of emotions that show up when we lose something or someone important.

How we experience life's losses is influenced by our history, cultural contexts, gender, roles, families of origin, and previous experiences. Grief and its many emotions can keep us off-kilter by mixing up our thoughts, emotions, and reactions in a never-ending loop; it's something only time, compassion, hard work, and the act of mourning can heal.

Mourning is different from grieving. Dr. Alan Wolfelt of the Center for Loss defines the difference like this:

> If grief is what we think and feel inside, what is mourning? Mourning is the outward expression of our grief.
>
> Mourning is crying, talking about the loss, journaling, sharing memories, and telling stories. Other ways to mourn include praying, making things, joining in ceremonies, and participating in support groups. Mourning is how, over time, we begin to heal. It's through active and honest mourning where we reconstruct hope and meaning in our lives.[20]

Grief is a natural human response to loss, filled with thoughts and emotions that are sometimes automatic and other times modelled and learned. Through the process of mourning, we can find helpful ways to express our grief, and learn how to integrate the loss into our lives so we can carry on. The integration of our losses is critical in finding healing and wholeness.

Mourning helps us to accept the reality of the impact of the loss and learn to live from a place of restoration. When we begin the process of restoration, we change. We can all be restored and transformed into something new, like the cherished broken bowls in the art of kintsugi. We are still the same people we know from before, but we're also different because of our loss and suffering. Loss changes us.

We have control over the way we choose to mourn, and we can learn new ways to mourn. It will be different for each of us, because we are different from one another and our circumstances, experiences, needs, past histories, and reactions are also different.

Grieving alone for long periods of time without engaging in the helpful and hopeful activities of mourning can cause us to get stuck. Through mourning we find ways in which to work through the impact of our loss. It helps us make sense of our emotions. It helps us see beyond the pain and suffering. It helps us investigate the next part of our story.

Mourning requires us to step out with courage, faith, and hope. We need courage to explore and feel the difficult, messy emotions and accept how they impact us. We need faith to trust in the unknowns surrounding us and in a God who promises to be with us and wants good to come from it. We need hope to believe in something bigger than us, our desires, and our experiences.

We place our hope in a good God, in the process, and in the healing we receive.

Mourning acts like a kind of scaffolding to help us integrate loss into our lives, finding new ways to embrace life, and not just survive but thrive. We come to learn how the loss and suffering changes us permanently, while at the same time seeing how it offers us opportunities to live from a place of acceptance and wholeness where we can see things more clearly, including the good and the difficult, and live in more meaningful and purposeful ways than before.

Articulating what I accept about my cancer experience has helped me to mourn. I accept that nothing I or anyone else did caused my cancer. I accept that no one knows why I ended up this way. It's not because I'm unlucky or that I've reached my expiration date; it's a reality that *just is*. There is much we don't know about our bodies. We don't always fully understand why some people develop cancer and others don't. It's a mystery. I accept this.

Cancer is the most difficult and challenging threat I've ever faced—and the challenges never really end because I continue to face side effects from surgery, radiation, and seeing my reflection in the mirror. Many interventions have been taken to save my life, but the results will always be with me, visible when I speak, eat blink, or swallow—or even when

I try to whistle while puttering around the house, forgetting that I can't whistle any longer.

These triggers serve as regular reminders. But I get to choose how I think about what these experiences mean to me.

Most recently, I've accepted how normal it is to feel constant tension or tightness in the areas of my body where I've endured surgical procedures or treatment; it would be unrealistic to expect otherwise.

So I have chosen to turn and pray, acknowledging the sadness and challenges of the loss but also extending prayers of gratitude. Gratitude for being alive. Gratitude for the surgeons who saved my life and continue to carefully watch my progress. Gratitude for the miracle of healing and wholeness and for how well I now feel. Gratitude for all the new opportunities I have received because of it. Gratitude for the adventure of writing this book.

It isn't helpful to dwell only on what I've lost because I can't change the past. I must also look forward to uncovering new opportunities along the way. In the process, I have learned to regularly gift myself with compassion and empathy, and to coach myself to brace against adopting a victim mentality. Shame can slip into my thinking from time to time, especially when a new struggle appears.

Many consider a cancer patient's journey to be over once they begin to act and look normal again. But it's never really over. Cancer treatment only marks the beginning. We carry the physical loss with us daily, because it happened not just to us but inside us as well. It affects us mentally, emotionally, and spiritually too. We will always be in a process of restoration because of the side effects of treatment that can show up years later, along with the ongoing need for self-care and self-monitoring in order to stay healthy for as long as possible. The threat of recurrence is ever before us.

My losses represent the beginning of my story.

The impact of the losses, along with the ongoing challenges of living an unknown future and choosing to live it well with trust and choosing to be fully alive one day at a time, identifies the middle of the story. This section is filled with fewer challenges and is infused with much hope and joy.

Yet the process of finding hope, wholeness, and joy is long and challenging. I will continue to pursue it through to the end of my story.

Grief Witnessed

By month ten of my recovery, I expect things to become easier, not harder. Why is this still so stinking hard?

Today is a bad day. Each new medical condition with which I'm diagnosed causes an increase in physical discomfort and pain. Everything hurts from the top of my head to the bottom of my toes.

"Just opening my eyes, blinking, opening my jaw, chewing, swallowing, moving my neck, wrists, fingers, spine, knees, and feet triggers physical aches and pains," I complain to my husband. "I can't get away from it."

Being wide awake at 4:30 a.m. is now a regular habit. I run through the mental checklist of what I need to stop doing and start doing instead.

Stop watching news before bed. Read for half an hour before sleeping rather than just ten minutes. Drink only one coffee per day, not two. If I wake up, I mustn't under any circumstances check my watch to find out the time. I should stop thinking so much and practice what I know works: breathe, relax, pray. Get rid of all the worry and clutter in my head. Just breathe, 1–2–3–4 in, and 1–2–3–4 out.

Environmental influences from the pandemic, isolation requirements, and the never-ending news about conflicts, surgical delays (especially for cancer patients), and the war in Ukraine triggers me emotionally. When the news comes on, I tear up at the sight or sound of others' suffering. I shut off the news and grab a book instead.

The combination of physical and emotional overstimulation weakens my resolve. The recent bad news is substantial: my newly acquired health conditions, the recent loss of a dear friend after a ten-year battle with cancer, the frightening news about the possibility of our newly expected grandchild not surviving birth, and my husband's worsening health, which I'll discuss further in the next chapter. We also had a flood in our basement that required months of restorative work. All this while also being barraged with repeated images of human suffering... it's too much to bear in such a short period of time.

I'm not doing well, I admit to myself. *I have no margin left. Maybe I need to talk to someone who understands. I need to make decisions and can't because I feel overwhelmed.*

I decide to ask for help and call to book an appointment with a psychologist who's experienced in working with cancer patients.

I dread talking to counsellors. I know what they'll ask and know what they're looking for. Worse yet, I compare what they do with what I'd do as a counsellor. I wonder, do all counsellor types think like me? After all, I'm a professional; I should know how to help myself, right? I don't really need help.

I realize that I don't like feeling vulnerable with anyone. I'll need to prepare for the appointment and all the questions that I know I'll be asked. Coffee in hand, I sit down after making the appointment and start to do the hard work I've been avoiding, even though the appointment is several weeks away.

But I can't wait weeks. I need help now. If I were a client, what would I have them do?

"Start by making a list of everything on my mind which causes me angst," the counsellor suggests. *"Then prioritize the list from the biggest impact to the smallest."*

I pull out my journal and write down all the crises which have occurred over the previous ten months. The list grows, and grows, and grows.

I gaze down at the twelve bulleted items neatly organized on the page. Twelve crises in ten months. Wow. That's a lot of stuff to deal with!

Looking at each one, I know that if I were to take a stress test, the impact scores for most of the crises would be high. Why not take the assessment so I'll know for sure? I rifle through my counselling resources for an assessment and quickly score it. Most of the items do, in fact, score high. No wonder I feel stressed!

Why didn't I see this before? I'm overwhelmed, overstimulated, and emotionally exhausted.

"Anyone would be," the counsellor remarks, returning to validate my experience.

It seems that validation works even if you validate on behalf of yourself. I can't help but chuckle. I guess that falls into the category of self-compassion.

Day by day, since I'm up bright and early anyway, I take the time to reflect on each crisis and its impact on me emotionally and physically. Then I look at its spiritual impact and explore its meaning in light of God's goodness, His purposes, and what this means to me. I challenge myself with questions about what I really believe. This type of reflection takes some time, but it's necessary time.

I rifle through my favourite inspirational books, including ones with liturgical prayers written out, which eliminates the need for me to articulate a prayer with my own limited words. I also take out my Bible, journal, and fountain pen. Eventually I empty all the angst out of my head and heart onto the paper. In this way, I try to understand and make sense of it—and find some meaning from it.

With each exercise, I feel lighter.

This process helps me to eliminate the clutter that's holding me back from healing and creates space for me to take the time I need to make important decisions. It helps me break free of anything that's keeping me stuck so I can embrace the things that keep me moving forward.

I question, explore, reflect, process, and pray—a lot. Along the way I uncover new insights and meaning. And I heal. My process of writing, reflection, and prayer are further strokes of gold gently brushed over the crevices created by overwhelming feelings. They help me gain new perspective despite the challenges.

I start this way every few days when I awaken early. As I do this work over a few weeks, I eventually decide that I no longer need to see the psychologist. I figure I'll just cancel the appointment. After all, I'm already on my way…

Just as quickly, I self-correct: *"You need to keep the appointment anyway—just to check in and be sure. It won't cost you anything to do a check-in. At least go to visit him once. You don't have to go again if it's not helpful. There's nothing to lose."*

I think about all the times I've told my clients that sometimes we need to be our own cheerleader so we can keep doing what's in our best interests.

I'm glad I keep the appointment. The psychologist normalizes all my cancer experiences and reactions. I'm not the only one to experience these symptoms, he explains. It seems that it's harder for some cancer patients to see images of human pain and suffering.

"You've experienced a lot of really difficult situations in the last several months," he says. "No wonder you feel overwhelmed."

I also need to make a relatively easy medical decision. It's been difficult, though, because I'm overcome with fear of the associated risks of sustaining more long-term nerve damage. I'd get stuck comparing my present stenosis to other experiences of back and nerve pain over the last ten years.

Sure, the risk is low, but there are risks with every medical intervention. Many questions kept arising. Am I willing to live with that risk if it were to happen? Is the risk worth taking for just a temporary fix? Are there any adjustments I can make to my lifestyle to help make the pain subside?

I explain my dilemma to the psychologist: fear from previous experiences is affecting my ability to make a confident decision.

He reminds me about something I previously knew but forgot.

"Avoidance causes anxiety," he says. "It makes things worse. But postponement with a plan is sometimes a very good thing as long as there is a plan. If there is no plan, it's not postponement. It's avoidance."

Wise words. I let them sink in.

On my way home, I decide to add another P-word to his suggestion. First comes postponement, then comes plan... and now comes *permission*. If I give my perfectionist self the permission to postpone a decision, it might be easier for me to develop a plan which creates some margin for me to make a non-emotional decision in my best interests. I'll think on it.

Our losses, when shared in safe community, allow for our suffering to be witnessed. We can receive hope from the simple act of someone bearing witness to our pain, validating the difficulty, because they're there with us in it.

My ways of mourning have evolved over the years. The process, although difficult and challenging, is a very healing process, but it requires time.

I've learned that I must be careful about where and in what I place my hope. I also must be careful about what I allow into my head and heart while also giving myself permission to honestly mourn. And I must cultivate courage and self-compassion, stepping into the process with faith and expectation that God will meet me as I process my grief.

I just need to take the first step.

There are benefits and drawbacks to being a counsellor going through her own cancer experience. Everyone assumes we know what to do and how to do it. Sometimes even we mistakenly think we don't need help. We teach techniques to help clients become more aware of emotions, process them, and find helpful new perspectives and approaches. And as counsellors, if we practice the same approaches we teach others, we end up doing it alone.

But this means our grief goes unwitnessed. This is the biggest lesson I've learned: grief needs to be witnessed in community, because it teaches us to be vulnerable and recognize that we need safe people in our circle too.

Having people around us teaches us about how closely we are connected to and need one another. Without this witness, it's easy to become overwhelmed by our circumstances. It can happen to any of us. Being alone in our overwhelming situation can cause us to lose our way, and in that place we can mistakenly convince ourselves that others don't understand. This can lead us into self-isolating and self-protecting behaviours. We may conclude that harm will come from exposing our vulnerability and needs.

> **...grief needs to be witnessed in community, because it teaches us to be vulnerable and recognize that we need safe people in our circle too.**

Instead we need to reach out to safe people for help to make sense of the overwhelm. Sharing, exploring, understanding, and naming our pain's impact brings us hope and strength to take the next steps.

Five Pillars to Process Grief

Grief is a universal experience, yet mourning is different for each person. We all need to figure out the process that's most helpful for us. No one person is an expert for another's experience with grief.

No one person is an expert for another's experience with grief.

I use five pillars to help me in my own process of grieving and mourning: sharing, sojourning, soul care, exploring longings, and making meaning and finding purpose.

This isn't a linear process; I often move back and forth between these pillars depending on what lays heaviest on my heart:

- **Sharing.** I try to find a safe way to unpack and explore whatever emotions and pain currently reside in my heart in an open and honest way, out loud, or in a journal to God, and eventually to a trusted, accepting, and mature person. Grief needs to be witnessed in caring, supportive community.

- **Sojourning.** I ask God to walk with me in my suffering and restore me. I also ask trusted others to sojourn with me, whether they be family, friends, or professionals. Asking for help is a sign of courage, not weakness, and it draws us into community where our stories can be witnessed.

- **Soul care.** I take time to choose helpful soul care activities to minister to my body, mind, and spirit as I heal. This may include quiet, solitude, rest, outdoor walks, being creative, and prayer, etc. to facilitate the reflection and healing process.

- **Exploring longings.** I take time to consider the meaning of the uncomfortably deep longings I have, especially during a time of crisis, for comfort, peace, and restoration. Maybe this is God wooing us to His heart because He is the ultimate guide, comforter, peace-giver, restorer, and healer.

- **Making meaning and finding purpose.** I consider what the loss means to me, what I appreciated about life before the loss occurred, what cherished memories I want to bring with me into the future, how I can better understand how the loss changes my perception of my identity, how I want the loss to change me for the good and make me a better person, what I have learned from the experience, and how I might be able to offer encouragement to others who are experiencing the same loss.

Whatever process we choose to follow needs to consider all the different parts of us—the mind (thinking and emotions), body, and spirit. Suffering affects all parts of us and its impact on all those parts needs to be processed and integrated as we step forward.

This is a challenging, soul-filled, full-bodied process. It requires that we become more open and willing to learn, grow, and embrace difficult emotions and truths about ourselves and our circumstances. It helps us to move toward healing and wholeness.

Moving Toward and Moving Away

When we're suffering or grieving, we tend to either move away from or toward people. Moving toward God first helps us lament with Him privately and honestly about the difficulty of our situation.

Taking a bit of time away from people can create space for solitude with God and to process, gain new understanding, heal, and recover. Yet we must also move into healthy community for support and care.

Sometimes there is danger in moving toward people too much, or too soon, especially if we expect them to save us from our pain. Setting unhelpful expectations or putting them on a pedestal sends the message that we're victims needing to be rescued. We aren't victims; we don't need rescuing. Granted, our situation may be difficult, but it may be more helpful for a fellow sojourner to walk along with us from time to time as a loving witness to our lived experience and pain.

Finding safe people is important in our healing. Sometimes they need to be invited to come alongside us. These are often the people who tend not to pursue you with their expertise or prying questions; instead they will bless you with their gentle, loving, accepting presence—if you invite them in. But most often they'll wait patiently to be asked. They never act as experts or push their way in. They'll humbly admit that they are on the same kind of healing path themselves. They will become equals as you explore together in discovering hope. Listening and learning from each other is reciprocal. No one is the expert.

When I started out, I wish I'd had someone to talk to who knew what it was like to have oral cancer, someone with whom I could turn to for answers.

Unfortunately, I didn't. But I did have a wonderful husband, great children, loving family members, and friends who frequently checked in on me. They sent me verses and words of encouragement, food, flowers, and even thoughtful gifts. Many invited me for walks and outings—spring, summer, fall, and winter. I had, and still have, amazing surgeons and doctors with open-door policies who care for me with great patience, kindness, and skill, patiently answering my questions at each appointment. I consider every one of them to be special sojourners, even now, and I am beyond grateful for each one.

Sojourners are just like the kintsugi artists who use their time, compassion, gentleness, and kindness to offer hope and healing from the many tiny cracks which come along with suffering.

We can be a sojourner to someone else even while we're on our own journey. We can make a call or send a quick email or text to encourage them and let them know we're praying for or thinking of them. This can bring us life, knowing that what we've learned can be transformed into words of loving encouragement for another.

There is also a danger in moving away from people too often, thinking that no one can help or no one understands us. This can cause us to lose contact with others and render us alone and isolated. We've all learned, through the pandemic, how important and life-giving it is to stay connected. When we self-isolate, it's often hard to reconnect again. We need connection to survive, thrive, heal, and become whole.

Either extreme—too much connection or too little—is unhelpful. We are responsible for our own emotions and responses. When we own them, they become golden opportunities to learn, transform, and grow in ways we never imagined. No one can take this path of suffering for us. It's ours to take. But we can take it in community too.

Healthy relationships are reciprocal ones in which we don't expect others to save us or feel obligated to carry our load for us. These are the people with whom we can be interdependent with good boundaries, listening, empathizing, sharing insights, and acting as a witness to one another as we sojourn together.

The experience of grief and pain isn't just something to be endured, but rather something that can be shared with others—because the burden is lighter when we support one another. When we help each other carry our burdens, the burden becomes lighter and makes us feel less alone. In these times, and in sharing our stories, others can find strength and hope in the next steps too.

Grief needs to be witnessed. And mourning activities which we choose in community allow for grief to be witnessed as we prepare to re-enter everyday life by choosing hope and wholeness.

———————

HIGHLIGHTS

Sharing our loss in safe community allows for our suffering to be witnessed. Hope comes from someone bearing witness to our pain. Something that was broken but truly restored is indeed more beautiful and valuable than it was in its original form.

Reflections

Consider What Keeps Us Stuck

- Reacting with grief alone, for the long-term, can keep us stuck when we don't engage in the helpful and hopeful healing activities of mourning.
- Without a witness in our grief, it's easy to become overwhelmed by our circumstances.

Consider What Brings Life

- Grieving is a process which helps us begin to accept the reality of the impact of the loss and learn to live from a place of restoration.
- Sharing our loss in safe community allows for our suffering to be witnessed.

Personal Reflection

- Try drawing your own kintsugi bowls. Let each bowl represent something you're grieving. Select one and take time to consider a small encouragement you have already received relating to the topic that represents healing you have received so far. What is one thing you are grateful for in this?
- What is one thing you can do to get connected with a healthy and supportive community that supports people dealing with grief and loss?

Chapter Six

REAL VALUE

"Real isn't how you are made," said the Skin Horse.
"It's a thing that happens to you. When a child
loves you for a long, long time, not just to play with,
but REALLY loves you, then you become Real."[21]
— Margery Williams

TAP-TAP-TAP GO my fingers. It's two o'clock in the morning and here I am, texting my husband.

I crane back my swollen neck one last time to scan the top of the hospital bed, trying to locate the nurses' button. I can't see it anywhere.

My courage wanes and my filter slips down another inch. My patience is completely gone. Where *is* that stupid thing? I need ice and a Tylenol to soothe the horrible pain in my throbbing head.

I am freezing cold and sleep is beyond my reach. Nurses are beyond my reach…

I'm a few days out from major surgery and look at my arm, the one still hooked up to an IV, then at the long food tube running into my nose and down into my stomach. The tube is tacked to the inside of my nostril with a stitch.

I examine the oxygen tube attached to the tracheostomy in my neck. The other arm sports a half-cast. Carefully tucked into bed hours earlier, pillows surround me, the safety sidebar securely raised. Once again, I cannot move.

No one can help me. I'm all alone to fend for myself. This is just too hard!

Feeling my discomfort rise, I consider my sorry predicament. I finally remember to breathe and reach for my phone to text my husband again. It's the middle of the night and I can't wait any longer.

I stare expectantly at my glowing screen. One minute passes. Two minutes pass. The only answer back is from the cursor. The *blink-blink-blink* faintly illuminates the room and all the nearby equipment.

My heart sinks. He's sound asleep.

I try calling, even though I can't speak. The phone rings and rings.

"Hello?" he answers groggily.

Tap-tap-tap. I tap my fingernail on the screen, feeling like a stupid woodpecker. He's gotta know it's me. *Tap-tap-tap.*

I hear deafening silence on the other end of the phone. Poor guy. He's half-asleep. I'm so selfish waking him.

"Hello? Hello?"

He's awake! My index finger, on the ready, goes *tap-tap-tap.*

He hangs up again. Ohhh, great.

The knot in my chest tightens a bit more. My fear shows up again, an unhelpful, unwanted, fairweather friend.

Motivated by pain and discomfort, I make a list in my head about how to solve my dilemma. What's the morse code for SOS? I shake my head at the absurdity of it.

Seriously, you're going nuts, I tell myself.

Part of me wants to laugh, part of me wants to cry. Discouragement wins. Feeling invisible, alone, and desperately in pain, my only recourse is tears. How can all this be happening?

Somehow, I pull myself together and attempt a second call to my husband, then a third. *Tap-tap-tap, tap-tap-tap.*

Finally! He answers, and this time he's awake enough to realize it's me. He reads my texts and responds.

He places a quick call to the nurses' station and a cheerful nurse immediately comes to the rescue.

Finally seen and heard, my needs addressed, I find rest for the remainder of the night. But not before carefully asking the nurse to pin the call button close to my hand.

Becoming Real

Unhelpful thinking can show up when we feel vulnerable, when we're hurting, and when we need help. It can result in falsely believing that we aren't seen and aren't important or heard. Worse yet, we feel abandoned. From this, we conclude there must be something wrong with us.

This kind of thinking can become a source of shame in times of crisis or suffering. And it starts with our thoughts. That which we believe about ourselves, our circumstances, and others can lead us into unhelpful thinking and emotions.

My own self-shaming messages regularly crept into different parts of my recovery because my face, neck, and tongue were swollen for months. On the surface, I thought I looked grotesque. I felt rather ugly, even though I knew my body was healing and learning new ways of operating. I just required a lot of time to heal.

My tongue needed to relearn how to eat and swallow, starting with thick beverages and then moving to puréed foods. From there, I tried soft-chew foods and eventually to anything else I wanted to try as long as I could avoid choking. I also needed to learn how to move the tongue in my mouth to pronounce words coherently.

Since certain lymph nodes were removed, I needed to learn how to move naturally occurring fluids out through other nodes through daily massaging. If not, my face would begin to swell uncomfortably.

In the early weeks, I desperately wanted to go back to normal, and I thought frequently about my losses. When I wasn't fearful about the future, discouragement moved in to keep me off-balance. I was often stuck between past longings and a fearful, unknown future.

Once I made the decision not to let cancer get the better of me, or make me feel like I wasn't good enough, or steal my joy, my attitude finally began to shift. I carefully listened to what I said to myself and where I put most of my attention—in the past, the present, the future, or fantasies. I was determined to shift my thoughts so they wouldn't affect my outlook. My mission was to eliminate any unhelpful thinking and do everything in my control to recover and become as strong and as healthy as possible.

I wanted to excel at speaking despite the surgery and tongue flap. My desire to speak as clearly as possible grew quickly.

As soon as I return home, I practice speaking. I dig out my old linguistics books from my English-as-a-second language days, thinking that my pronunciation resources might help. Day-by-day, with mirror in hand, I review where I need to place my tongue to pronounce different sounds and words. I form words backward, syllable by syllable, until I can clearly pronounce a complete word.

I do this over and over. The practice can't hurt, and it just might help.

I also faithfully perform strengthening exercises. I pull the tongue up and way back to allow the tip of my tongue to manoeuvre itself against my teeth. This is the hardest part because it's an unnatural position and somewhat tiring. But before long, the sounds coming out of my mouth grow clearer. I progress and practice forming strings of sounds, words, and sentences—forward and backward—as well as tongue twisters. I want to be coherent.

I video my efforts, becoming my own student; I pretend I'm listening to someone else as I evaluate my progress. I'm quite thankful that I taught pronunciation classes years ago while in graduate school.

At first, the effort it takes to pronounce each syllable makes the flow of my speech choppy and slow. I realize this will affect my listeners' comprehension. Our ears expect a certain musical rhythm to our words, which requires us to place the proper stress on the right syllables.

But each day of painstaking practice brings improvement.

I never knew that tongues could get tired, but I reason that reading longer sentences might help with this. Out comes one of my grandkid's books, *The Velveteen Rabbit*. If I can read this, I will be able to read to the grandchildren online. It's a weekly activity we started during the pandemic when we couldn't visit one another, but with my limited speech my husband had to take on the role as reader while I became the page turner.

The Velveteen Rabbit is a lovely story about a stuffed toy rabbit who was given to a little boy one Christmas morning. I muster up the energy to read the story aloud. I flip open the book to a random page and begin to read:

> "Real isn't how you are made," said the Skin Horse. "It's a thing that happens to you. When a child loves you for a long, long time, not just to play with, but REALLY loves you, then you become Real."
>
> "Does it hurt?" asked the Rabbit.
>
> "Sometimes," said the Skin Horse, for he was always truthful. "When you are Real you don't mind being hurt."
>
> "Does it happen all at once, like being wound up," he asked, "or bit by bit?"
>
> "It doesn't happen all at once," said the Skin Horse. "You become. It takes a long time. That's why it doesn't often happen to people who break easily, or have sharp edges, or who have to be carefully kept. Generally, by the time you are Real, most of your hair has been loved off, and your eyes drop out and you get loose in the joints and very shabby. But these things don't matter at all, because once you are Real you can't be ugly, except to people who don't understand." [22]

As I read the story, I realize that I'm still feeling more than a little sorry for myself, not really seeing how God can use my walk with cancer for good while also transforming me in the process. I'm hopeful, though, because I believe He can.

But I'm also filled with doubt because I can't see the possibility that my situation is anything other than just plain bad. I feel ugly, scarred, bruised, swollen, and incoherent, all while sporting a droopy eye and a crooked mouth which, in a most unbecoming way, sometimes drools. All I can see are the negatives.

I feel shabby and unlovable, like the little rabbit in the story. Somehow I realize that I'm no longer the *me* I knew anymore. I regularly catch myself falling into a victim mindset and wonder who'd ever really want me or want to be with me looking and sounding like this.

I begin reading to my husband, forgetting that I had asked him to inconspicuously videotape me so I could have a record of what I sound like after the surgery. Oblivious to the recording, I read the exchange between the bunny and horse, blinking back tears. I hear my own voice read out these impactful words while one hand holds the book and the other securely pushes the side of my mouth into the middle of my face to help me enunciate. I choke up with tears.

I had forgotten about this video until I came across it a year after my radiation treatments ended. I cherish the short clip now because it's a good reminder of when I realized that despite the fact that different parts of me were lopped off, disfigured, loose, or droopy, I might become more real along the way. Just like the little bunny. I'd become a more real version of myself—different, but more real. More *me*.

This is the opportunity and adventure with which I've been presented. In the beginning, I thought it a bit strange to think like this, but as I reflected on the idea I recognized it as a biblical concept. Suffering has a way of transforming us, stripping away all of our masks and helping us become more real as we live well. God made us to be whole and helps us reclaim wholeness in our lives—if we're open to it.

As a counsellor, I spent years helping clients find ways to become more authentic, releasing unhelpful false identities and welcoming in the parts they had let slip away over time due to distractions, work, pressures, relationships, or busy schedules. These clients would transform before my very eyes, blossoming and growing and healing. I had always considered this transformation a miracle and a privilege to witness.

Transformation for them. Transformation for me. Transformation for you.

And so in this children's book I was reminded that to be real and whole, we need to remember that God originally created us to be whole and real. But none of us stay in this original form because of the impact of this world, our experiences, our choices, and other people's choices. Yet God enables us to reclaim our original identity and uses our experiences, especially the difficult ones, to help us find out what's truly real about us and offers opportunities to release that which is not.

As we become open to what we can learn and how we can grow, no matter how difficult it may appear, the great biblical mystery of redemptive transformation helps us become more real too. More ourselves. More of who we were originally made to be. It can become an avenue into wholeness, for we were designed to be whole.

This is a sacred journey, and we are all invited to take it.

Crossroads as Sacred Places

The little story about the rabbit helped me realize I was measuring my value by the external, observable parts of myself without considering my true internal value. The shame I felt about how I looked and sounded was unhelpful, especially since I was still healing and had been assured by many that it wouldn't always be this way.

Thus began a critical examination of the things I was letting into my mind, things that influenced how I saw myself and therefore impacted my healing.

Years ago, I offered psychoeducational sessions on shame resilience using Brené Brown's curriculum *Connections*.[23] The program explains that when we can't achieve or maintain the expectations we have about ourselves or others have on us—like who we should be, how we should be, or what we should be—we can experience shame, feeling like we aren't enough and that there's something wrong with us. She defines shame this way: "Shame is the intensely painful feeling or experience that we are flawed and therefore unworthy of connection or belonging."[24]

As a person of faith, I have come to see shame as an unhelpful influence along the path toward becoming whole, becoming real. In my faith tradition, we believe that our image comes from God because of who He is, whether we accept it or not—whether we believe or not. God sees and accepts everyone as His child, and each of us are made in His image. He creates good things. He created the world; He created us. We are of value because of who He is, not because of anything we've ever done or can do. He creates our value, not anyone or anything else.

Understanding our value this way is very freeing because we don't have to earn it through our worth, status, education, income, looks, social connections, or any other reason. This doesn't mean we can't be ambitious, working with all we are and all we have or strive for excellence; it just means we already have value. We don't need to work hard to gain value, which can be a vicious cycle when the bar we're reaching for just keeps rising.

When we allow cultural and familial expectations to influence how we see ourselves, we can slip into living from a false identity. Not to mention how exhausting it is to maintain. No one is immune from this, no matter how well we think we understand our value. The continual onslaught of mixed messages can blind us from seeing the truth.

When we burn out, go through a crisis, suffer in some way, or have our external sources of value stripped from us, we come face to face with a crisis of belief.

For me, after my surgery, I had lots of thoughts. Do people only see the cancer patient label when they look at me? Will they avoid me? Do I elicit pity or discomfort in others? Can I speak publicly anymore? How can I make jokes and quip now that my brain and speech seem slower? Will I be able to form my words quick enough? Will I still have value as a professional now that I have a speech impediment? Can I still teach? Can I facilitate groups? Will I ever be asked to speak again?

I also wondered whether certain groups would accept me. After all, I know that gender and age surely do affect who's in and who's out. What about a cancer diagnosis? Or some other type of loss or suffering?

Cynicism crept into my thinking.

What I sometimes forget is that when others look at us, they see through a biased lens, and their bias will be influenced by a variety of factors including their own experiences, family, and culture. Instead of seeing each other as God does, as good enough, we make presuppositions—and these views often lead us into a place of judgment if we don't intentionally become aware of our thought processes.

Judgment can become a type of automatic, dualistic thinking. We judge what's good or bad, what's right or wrong, without any awareness of the biases that influence us. But dualistic presuppositions don't look for any other possible way to be; it's just opinion and judgment. Sometimes there *are* clear rights and wrongs, of course. I'm not referring to those times. I'm referring to the kind of judgmental thinking which brings shame into our relationships instead of emulating love and acceptance for people's suffering.

I've already discussed how dualistic thinking causes us to only recognize black versus white, right versus wrong. Non-dualistic thinking creates room for other options, maybe even some mystery, allowing us to cultivate curiosity, empathy, and understanding for one another instead of judgment. We become more welcoming and hospitable toward one another, more willing to learn.

It's not about what we do or what others have done to us that makes us feel shamed or devalued. Rather, shame comes from what we choose to think about, believe, and take on. We can't control or change other people's reactions, but we can change how we think about them.

It's simple. Accepting judgments sounds like this: *If they're right, then I'm wrong. Maybe there is something wrong with me.* This is shame speaking. Yet if we become curious enough to try to understand the lens through which another person sees us, we might learn more about their beliefs instead of taking that shame onto ourselves as part of our identity.

When someone shames us, it's not about us. It's about the lens the other person is using. Sometimes people shame others to feel better about themselves. It comes from a place of brokenness, fear, or misinterpretation. Or even false belief. When we remain curious in our discomfort, we can avoid accepting shame and avoid reciprocating it back onto others. We are called to love, not to judge or shame. When we shame others, we shame ourselves.

One participant in a shame resiliency group I led years ago described what being shamed felt like for her. She said it was like someone throwing a thick black gooey blanket of slime over her so the other person could no longer see the other good parts of her. The experience rendered her invisible. She said that she took on the shame label others assigned to her. Yet the truth is that we are more than what others think or say about us.

This image of being slimed has always stuck with me, because if the blanket of shame covers us then the valuable parts of who we are, the person God created us to be, can no longer be perceived. We somehow become the judgment and label attributed to us, and that label is all people see. But shame never, ever tells the truth.

...shame never, ever tells the truth.

When we're suffering, shame is the last thing we need on the way to becoming whole. It hides our real value, even from ourselves.

Contradictions at the Crossroads

What about us? How do we know if we're accidentally shaming ourselves or others? One easy thing to look for is contradictions between our thoughts and behaviours. When contradictions show up between what we supposedly believe and what we do, we may be believing something untrue.

Others can shame us, and we can shame ourselves, by placing an unwanted label on our physical, emotional, or social condition. A divorce? You're a divorcée. Death of a spouse? You're a widow or widower. Job loss? You're unemployed. Substance abuse? You're an addict. Cancer patient? You're a cancer victim. These are all negative labels, and they bring shame. When we wear these labels, people only see the circumstance that happened to us and ignore all the other parts. This is judgment, and it sentences us to believing lies.

These lies aren't who we are. Labels we receive into our heart and mind that objectify or devalue us can profoundly influence our direction in life. When we label and shame others or ourselves, it becomes a sentence of rejection and isolates us from healing communities—and those communities are such an important component of healing.

Shame or Pride?

One winter morning, while still struggling with so many physical changes, I come across an online article about a mother's reflection over her little girl being born with some deformities.[25] The piece helps me gain insight about the labels we place on ourselves. She writes about the first time she met her daughter. She says that she was at a crossroads about how to move forward—would she move forward with shame about how her daughter looked or move forward with pride?

I confidently think to myself that if this were my child, I'd choose pride.

Suddenly a new challenging thought comes to me: *Yes, and what about for yourself? Shame or pride?*

Convicted, I let this question settle in and I slowly realize that I'm standing at my own crossroads right now. I can hold on to labels and be embarrassed about why people think I developed cancer, or about how I look, or feel ashamed of my speech impairment or long ugly scars. Or I can move forward with pride, even if I'm different than I was before. Different does not necessarily mean it's bad.

It's funny how we can think we really know something, but then a new challenge creates an opportunity that invites us to rethink what we thought we once knew, in order for us to know it more surely and deeply.

I remind myself that because I have value, I'm good enough. I'm learning to be the real me with all my new limitations. Because that's good enough.

The pep talk continues as I look for errors in my thinking processes. A lot of them seem to be surfacing. I need to look for the opportunity in these challenges and keep my eyes open for all the little blessings along the way, feeling grateful for what I have right now and for the time I have on earth. I remind myself that God is good, despite our circumstances. He can redeem every single bit of suffering, and along the way I can find hope and wholeness. I must learn to embrace the life I have.

> **...a new challenge creates an opportunity that invites us to rethink what we thought we once knew, in order for us to know it more surely and deeply.**

I have so much to be grateful for. There is a lot of good in my life, and many good people. How do I want to move forward? With shame or pride? Coming to a crossroads is an opportunity for change. We must choose which way to go.

A verse comes to mind:

> *Stand at the crossroads and look; ask for the ancient paths,*
> *ask where the good way is, and walk in it, and you will*
> *find rest for your souls.* (Jeremiah 6:16)

I long for rest for my soul. Not just for now, but also in the future. Most importantly, I need to remember that a diagnosis or invasive operation doesn't change who I am—nor does it change my heart, spirit, or soul. It especially doesn't change my unique value as a person.

With time and reflection, I've come to accept the parts of my journey that are a gift and see each of them as a type of miracle. Surgery and treatment have helped me stay alive. They don't make me any less me. I'm grateful for that. After all, it's just my physical body, and if my appearance or speech changes, it doesn't change the essence of who I am—because of Whose I am.

I've spent countless years with clients reflecting on their identity and reminding them that we aren't what others think about us, what we experience or feel, and what others have done to us. That's shame speaking.

And as I said before, shame never, ever tells the truth.

When shame speaks untruths, it blinds us. We can't see what's true and real. We're good enough and of great value no matter what others think, no matter what they say, no matter what has happened to us, and no matter what others have done to us.

Redemptive Thinking

Being a person of faith helps me to process the idea of suffering through a redemptive lens—a lens which helps me hold firmly to my identity and make sense of my own story in the context of God's bigger story of redeeming the world to Himself. There is purpose in everything, and He can transform anything to have purpose.

It's easy to forget this when we're tired and not looking after our own self-care, including soul care. We can feel victimized and end up judging others. This is when doubt seeps in and leads us into a path of overwhelm. It's a vicious cycle which results in more pain.

Only when we take a step back, pull away, and reflect in solitude and prayer can we gain new insight into how God might use our experiences in the bigger picture He has designed for us.

As we remember and remind ourselves of who we are and what we believe, we can find comfort, peace, hope, and strength to keep persevering under intense loss, struggle, and pain.

A Crossroads Conversation

Morning coffee times are special at our home—slow, quiet, sacred times. Sometimes my husband and I just read and share tidbits of interest. Other times we chat as we enjoy and embrace a slower pace of life. Even our dog knows not to pester us. Mostly she rests quietly as we start our day. When she wants something, she comes up and leans against my leg, gently asking for attention.

Sitting across from my husband one morning, I explain what I'm coming to learn as I recover and adjust from surgery and treatment.

"I'm learning to embrace all the unknowns about *why* I developed cancer and all the ambiguity around it," I explain. "It helps when I can shift my focus from the unknowns to focus on what I know to be true and on hopeful ways of thinking, even when I don't know what the future will hold..."

When someone is faced with a type of cancer with a high recurrence rate, one which might bring more suffering and disfigurement, or an earlier than anticipated death, the challenge is not in dying. The challenge is in living. It comes down to me choosing to live well in the midst of all the messiness and learn to trust. It's about embracing the life we're living right now with all the joys, challenges, and limitations. The choices I make bring life. There are no guarantees for any of us. Dying is a universal reality. We all need to figure out for ourselves what we believe, because eventually we'll all die someday—and none of us know the timing of our last day.

My beliefs and my faith sustain me, giving me confidence in God's promises. The hardest part is being committed to choosing to live well on a daily basis and embracing hope without becoming distracted or overwhelmed by the unexpected circumstances that crop up.

I must choose to live well now, in the present, with joy and hope. The hardest part is knowing how to be fully alive and thrive when I don't know if the cancer will return or if I'll need to face more surgery or treatment. Because of this, I have a growing desire not to waste any time, because I don't really know how much time I have left.

I'm also reminded that I'm not the only one dealing with health issues in our home. Just a few months earlier, during a routine check and angiogram, my husband met a cheerful, keen doctor who was new to our local hospital. The doctor confidently explained that he could remove several blockages which other doctors hadn't been able to five years earlier when they were first detected. He had previously endured three failed attempts at putting in stents, and over the years his health had slowly declined. We knew he was on borrowed time. If one of his arteries were to burst, there would be no way for him to survive it.

After several hours of a special procedure to remove the calcified blockages, this new doctor was successful! Several months later, my husband felt like a new man—clear-minded, energetic, active, and cheerful. He too has been given a miraculous gift of health.

Over coffee, I ask about his recent experience with heart disease and how he had dealt with not knowing what would happen to him. He had lived with *not knowing* for five years!

"What has helped me the most is to learn to live in the present," he says. "It's really about being present, in the moment, with gratitude for what I have and to not worry about the future."

We've both learned to cultivate intentional choices every day to be more present, to trust, and to embrace hope. This brings life to our souls instead of allowing worry or fear to produce death.

Amidst suffering and sorrow, the invitation to embrace our real value allows us to receive that which is true and helpful about ourselves and to release that which is not—despite what we've lost, how we look, what we do for a living, how sick, disfigured, poor, or lonely we feel, or even how sad or fearful we feel about our circumstances. That which we let into our hearts eventually comes out in our thinking, decisions, and actions toward ourselves, others, and even God. It's what we carry with us until we find ways to allow it to change us and help us become whole and real.

In a crisis, we can easily begin to believe untrue things, especially if we have a habit of jumping to conclusions or using other kinds of unhelpful thinking styles.

Embracing life means acknowledging that we're only finite humans and we need each other in our various communities and times of need to thrive, support, and love one another. In this way, we facilitate transformation, becoming more of who we were meant to be and taking steps toward becoming real.

Author Timothy Keller writes about how suffering can make us a better or worse person, and how God uses suffering to transform our attitudes toward ourselves and others.[26] He writes about how God helps us examine ourselves when the worst arises to show us our weaknesses. Ultimately, this whole experience can strengthen our walk with God. Keller writes, "Nothing is more important than to learn how to maintain a life of purpose in the midst of painful adversity."[27]

Becoming real helps us take more steps and gain clarity about our identity, weaknesses, and purpose. Walls come down and our false identities crumble, revealing our true identities.

As we step into this process with curiosity, courage, and faith, we become more real because suffering often drives us toward God. And when we allow ourselves to be fully loved by God and others, while also placing our faith and trust in His goodness and ultimate plan for our lives, our attitudes and perspectives change.

HIGHLIGHTS

Suffering has a way of changing us, helping us to become more real as we walk through life. God made us to be whole and helps us reclaim that wholeness—if we're open to it. God has a way of being able to use our lives to help us find out what's real and offers opportunities to release that which is not.

Reflections

Consider What Keeps Us Stuck

- Unhelpful thinking can show up when we feel vulnerable, are hurting, and need help.
- Others can shame us, and we can shame ourselves by placing unwanted labels on our physical, emotional, and social conditions.
- Shame never, ever tells the truth.

Consider What Brings Life

- We were designed to be whole.
- We should cultivate curiosity, empathy, and understanding for one another instead of judgment.
- We can't control or change other people's reactions, but we can change how we think about them.

Personal Reflection

- What is one unhelpful false label you have given yourself or others have given to you? What one thing gets overlooked about your unique design when that label is used on you?
- Journal your answer: "When I'm labelled with _____, people don't see _____ about me." What one thing are you grateful for about your unique design?

Chapter Seven

CULTIVATE RESILIENCE

The most important thing in your life is not what
you do; it's who you become. That's what you'll
take into eternity.[28]

—Dallas Willard

WE BECOME BETTER ABLE to deal with adversity through the resilience-
building activities we faithfully practice. When we look at the word
resilient, we can see that it means "bouncing back from difficulties."[29]

We are often pushed into a crisis without any kind of experience
or preparation; we end up stumbling through our period of suffering
with shocked surprise. The worst emerges from us rather than the best.
We get through, but not always unscathed. And bouncing back may be
harder than expected.

But what if?

What if we become better prepared—body, mind, and spirit—and
therefore more resilient? What if we make the choice to live well in the
next part of our story? What if we manage our expectations that keep us
stuck? What if we find ways to embrace life and the concept of wholeness,
persevering along the way and mourning our losses? What if we become
the best version of ourselves? What if we become more real because of our
value?

Some crises we take in stride; others feel like never-ending traumas,
rendering us helpless or even hopeless. Building up our emotional,

physical, and spiritual resilience helps us become better at coping with crises more productively.

Many people use denial, distractions, or numbing out to avoid dealing with difficult situations for fear of pain and suffering. How we meet difficult challenges depends on many things: our personality, preferred style of doing things, learned habits of mind, learned behaviours, previous experiences, and existing level of resiliency.

Considering my surgeon once told me that our bodies are designed to heal, it makes perfect sense to me that the whole of God's original design for us is geared toward healing. God never wastes anything we experience. Our crises can be used to transform us. Our part is to remain open and participate in the process, knowing that we will discover a more authentic way to live as we grow and transform.

Therefore, we must consider what attitudes, skills, and methods need to be cultivated to increase our ability to deal with adversity. When practiced and strengthened, we can use these tools to nurture healing within us. Let's consider some of these tools so that we grow and thrive, not just survive.

Creating Margin to Cultivate Resiliency

We prepare for the journeys on which we embark, whether they be road trips, exotic vacations, or outings in nature. We prepare because we want these trips to be safe, enjoyable, and successful.

We research our destination and make plans. We identify potential risks, then make schedules and reservations. We pack intentionally, ensuring we won't become hungry or overtired. Sometimes we even invite others along to avoid being on our own.

Despite the most intricate plans, the unexpected still can and does happen. However, the time we invest in planning isn't lost. Being well-equipped at the outset of a journey makes later adjustments much easier. These preparations form a critical scaffolding that create space, or margin, to allow for alternative plans, avoiding the chaos that can make a journey so unpleasant.

If this is true for recreational journeys, shouldn't the same kind of margin be available for difficult journeys? Why do we tend not to invest the same amount of energy and preparation for life's challenging journeys?

Creating margin is the practice of leaving enough room or space in our minds and hearts to face challenges without becoming overwhelmed or developing unhealthy or harmful coping behaviours. This requires time and commitment to learn about and attend to our inner needs, thoughts, and emotions. When we do this before a crisis hits, we develop skills that can help when one does.

Finding margin is like an athlete preparing for a marathon. They build up their strength and balance their lives with healthy food, rest, and restoration. They practice their skills to improve their strength and endurance. They find a coach to equip them, and they listen to the coach's advice. The race may still challenge the athlete, but they fare better due to their preparation. Cultivating these healthy habits ensures they will be sustained throughout the race and be able to make adjustments to meet new needs as they unfold.

Intentional preparation builds a safety net of margin. Through this practice, we become more resilient and able to respond to the necessary changes we face.

A Surprise

Twenty years ago, I took my mother to England for a dream mother/daughter trip. During this memorable trip, I learned firsthand how preparation helps.

Every aspect of our trip was planned out, mostly by me, because I wanted things to go smoothly so we could create wonderful memories together.

Unwittingly, I made some faulty assumptions.

My mother gave birth to me late in life, making her older than most of my friends' mothers. She was eighty-two at the time of our trip, but as spry and sharp as they come. Mom, now gone for more than ten years, was a retired nurse. She was a friendly, generous-hearted woman and had the greatest smile ever. She was a fun traveling companion. She loved to explore and was always up for an adventure.

When the big day arrived, we said our goodbyes and caught our flight. Everything went according to plan. We soon arrived at Heathrow Airport, made our way to the car rental office, and climbed into our car. We were in London, England, so of course I had fully prepared to drive on the right-hand side. I was excited to drive from the other side of the car, being left-handed. I helped my mom into the passenger seat and hopped into the driver's seat.

One thing I hadn't prepared for was my mother's reaction. While planning for the trip, she had cheerfully agreed to be the navigator. Settling in, I handed her the map on which I had painstakingly highlighted all the routes we were to take. She lifted up the map, peered at it, leaned forward, wiggled her glasses closer to her eyes and pushed them up the bridge of her nose with her index finger and thumb. She squinted, long and hard.

My eyes widened in wonder. I froze in my seat as I watched the event unfold in slow motion. She turned the map left, turned it right, then flipped it upside-down and back again. At last she dropped the map in her lap and sweetly twisted her body to face me.

"Which way does this blasted thing go?" she asked with some exasperation.

More than slightly stunned, I blinked a few times and realized that this woman had absolutely no clue how to read a map. Worse yet, she couldn't even see it. My index finger slowly rubbed the skin under my left eyebrow as I tried to stifle the laughter bubbling up deep inside me. It was a nervous kind of laughter filled with sheer, unadulterated fear.

The reality of our situation slowly sank in. In slow motion, I reached across the stick shift, picked up the map, and folded it neatly. My future flashed before my eyes. I was on my own to navigate for the next nineteen long days. What was I going to do?

I smiled. "It's okay, Mom, I'll be fine. I can do it myself. It's all good."

Forced by this new adjustment, I took some additional time every morning of the trip to study the map. I memorized key landmarks and frequently pulled over to update myself on the directions, even though I used the excuse that we had to stretch our legs.

In the end, we made our way around without too much difficulty, but not without a few shrill screams of laughter as we tore through certain roundabouts more than once, trying to read signs and find the right exit to take. We only became lost once, and only once did I accidentally enter a parking lot on the wrong side.

I still chuckle about this trip and all the detours we took as we drove around, despite the extra bit of stress and adjustments we had to make. In the end, it was worth it. We had a wonderful time and I built beautiful memories with my wonderful mother I will cherish for years to come.

Effort Is an Investment

Despite careful preparation, things can still go awry—but the invested effort is still of value because the preparation creates new skills and ways of thinking, helping us to get through a crisis without getting overwhelmed. We can bounce back and adjust to difficult situations. Preparation also builds confidence and readiness. Investing in any kind of preparation creates a foundation from which we can build new attitudes, skills, and methods to strengthen body, mind, and spirit.

In order to find ways to create margin in our lives, we need to know ourselves and what our needs are—body, mind, and spirit. We must also consider who will best guide us and cheer us on.

Investing time in preparation before a crisis strikes gives us the necessary margin to develop new ways of thinking and processing issues, caring for ourselves, and problem-solving. It helps us make room in our heads and hearts to learn new ways to regulate our emotions and gain new perspectives and insight. Having margin means we can rid ourselves of what is unhelpful and receive what is helpful for every part of us. Without margin, it's easy to become overwhelmed, especially if many difficult experiences strike in a short timeframe. We are only human, and we have limits.

The preparation we choose will help strengthen the soul, body, and spirit. Any heart and soul preparation we invest in now will help sustain us along the way when things do go awry.

Resilience as a Way of Life

Any type of soul preparation that's designed to build margin and build resilience in us is something that I'd call a soul care practice. For me, soul care practices have four common components, and their goal is to cultivate a way of life that brings wholeness.

Here are the four components:

- Receiving in
- Reaching up
- Reflecting and releasing
- Reaching out

Each of these components come with many practical exercises.

Receiving in. During this time, I often practice a meditative breath prayer or read a psalm or some other kind of contemplative prayer to help centre myself. This always brings peace and helps me release nagging thoughts or stresses currently on my mind.

I breathe in hope, love, and truth. I breathe out fear, anxiety, and unhelpful thinking.

Deep breathing helps me to focus and be present and aware of what bothers me. It prepares my heart to release my deeper concerns or worries and prepares me to welcome more hopefulness.

Reaching up. I usually start this time by praying. Then I read a small passage of Scripture, chosen from a prayer guide I have used for many years. It's a beautifully bound yearly calendar that identifies passages pertaining to many topics. With this guide, I don't have to figure out what I should read each day. Each week has a theme, followed by seven days of the week filled with reflective paragraphs to consider. Remarkably, the theme is usually what I need to read and hear.

The encouragement from this prayer time brings me hope, because it reminds me of God's goodness and His larger redemptive purposes.

Reflecting and releasing. Then I sit quietly, waiting for what comes to my mind. If I've been neglectful with my soul care, sometimes a busy to-do list floats through my preoccupied mind and I spend time releasing it all. I call this letting go of my clutter.

Other times, when my spirit feels quieter, a single thought, concern, or emotion might bubble up into my mind. If it's the busy list, I refocus on my breathing; if it's a concern of some kind, I talk to God about what's on my heart.

Sometimes talking is just a heartfelt prayer. Other times, especially when I feel a little emotional, I journal to ensure that my concerns aren't stuck rolling around in my head, causing me more angst once I'm done.

And sometimes nothing comes up. When that happens, I express my thankfulness for what I'm learning along the way. Each time is different.

This quiet time allows for a wonderful release that always lightens the load, bringing insight and new perspectives.

Reaching out. The reaching out process is twofold. It includes asking my community for help when I have a need and offering support to others if and when I'm able to help.

Asking for support is the hardest part for me. Admittedly it doesn't happen very often. As a person who has dedicated her life to helping others, it's not easy to be the one needing care. If I do speak up and ask for help, it most likely means I'm at my wit's end. It means I'm desperate, because I'm more likely to try to figure things out on my own and consequently leave the matter until I have no other choice but to ask for someone I implicitly trust to help.

Since my diagnosis, I've come to realize that I need to ask for help more often. When I take the chance and let my walls come down, the version of myself who emerges is a more real and more vulnerable person. The real me. This happens every single time when the person I reach out to shows kindness and compassion for me. They do it because they are safe, and they sincerely care for my well-being.

Community is a place where inner healing can happen. It's a place where we are surrounded by safe people who can tolerate being uncomfortable as they witness our challenges with patience, kindness, and love while gently encouraging us and keeping us pointed in the right direction in times of weakness. These people in my trusted circle include family, close friends, my pastor, my family doctor, and my surgeon—all people who care, support, encourage, and cheer me on in challenging times. I consider them all gifts from God.

This is my healing community. Here I can choose to release control. I don't have to protect my image of needing to have it all together. Here, I can choose to connect instead of withdraw—choose to be vulnerable rather than pretend to be strong.

Asking for help in community can bring hope and healing.

Supporting others is important too. During the first year after my surgery, I had several friends and family members who needed support during their own crises; their lives didn't stop just because I was in my own crisis.

Even in our own difficult situations, it can be greatly life-giving to reach out a supportive hand through simple acts of love, whether that be prayer, texts, calls, walks, making a meal, baking cookies, or babysitting children. In difficult times, we can empathize with the plight of others, recognizing that we all have moments of need—and we all need to be there for each other.

Soul Care Practices

The soul care practice of taking time to become quiet can raise our awareness of the myriad of thoughts, emotions, and reactions within us. It gives us time to attend to our needs emotionally, spiritually, and even physically. It's an investment of time that helps us become aware of the barriers inhibiting us from being our best selves. My best me. Your best you. And as we attend to the issues raised, our body, mind, and spirit heal, becoming more fully integrated. We become more whole and better able to see and embrace the hope before us.

Soul care practices are helpful in quieting our souls and helping us find ways to remove the clutter. They help us discover the kind of hope we seek.

What's a soul care practice? I've heard them referred to variously as a rule of life, a spiritual discipline, or a personal liturgy. There are many ways to describe daily habits and rituals we regularly practice to care for our soul. The common denominator is that they're all designed to cultivate a rich spiritual life. We aren't talking about creating a checklist of activities; it's more of a sustainable practice we undertake faithfully, like brushing our teeth a few times daily because it's a good self-care practice. Neglecting our oral care impacts our oral health. Soul care is no different. Neglect can create distance in us from God, others, and ourselves.

My favourite soul care practices help me draw closer to God no matter the circumstances I face. They help me take time to uncover ways to find balance, new perspectives, insights, peace, hope, and wholeness.

Finding the best practices for ourselves requires careful thought, exploration, and maybe even creating a guide that can be updated as we learn more about what works best and is sustainable. It requires thinking about how we might prepare for any difficulties ahead. We can consider different events that might happen over time and imagine what our souls might need to help us cope and sustain us through loss and suffering.

These activities help us develop simple easy-to-maintain habits that when practiced faithfully become a way of life. Therefore, when days of suffering eventually come, sometimes again and again, we'll have developed a muscle of spiritual resilience that helps us to thrive without losing hope along the way.

These regular practices hone our ability to become more aware of what hinders and helps us on a daily basis or what might be a barrier to our walk of faith.

Soul care practices can be nurtured and grown through a combination of activities, whether it be learning to identify, label, and express our emotions safely; discovering environments that make us feel whole; or cultivating opportunities for quiet time, prayer, and journalling, etc. that build inner soul strength and resilience. These practices help us learn to be as holistically healthy as we can and find ways to cope.

I have outlined some of my favourite practices in Appendix A.

Soul Care Starts by Cultivating Curiosity

If you're anything like me, my first tendency is to rail against injustices and any form of unkindness. It just seems so wrong, so unfair.

Many of us perceive our crises as unfair too. Yet maintaining a solely negative perception about our circumstances in the long-term, even as circumstances change, can keep us stuck in a cycle of negativity—that is, if we don't manage our perceptions over time. What we focus on can impact us. For example, it can affect what we feel in our body, or think in our mind, and influence our behaviours, health, relationships, and spirit, just to name a few.

What if we became curious instead and implemented new strategies to navigate through our various challenges? What we choose to think can help us become more resilient. Our response won't take the crisis away, or the pain, but it may help us cope and recover better as we cultivate ways to embrace life and hope.

And in so doing, when we look back at these difficult experiences, we will see them as a time during which we built unexpected strengths. We grew, changed, and became stronger—more resilient—coping in new ways without minimizing the losses that occurred.

When we cultivate curiosity, we gain new perspectives.

When we cultivate curiosity, we gain new perspectives. It starts with asking helpful questions related to all our parts—body, mind, and spirit. Formulating helpful questions leads us to discern our own specific needs.

In the coming pages, I will list my favourite questions. Take some time to consider them and create your own set of questions. The questions that come to your mind may be different, of course, because they'll be context-specific and based on your own needs.

1. Body. We are embodied souls and much of what we experience can and does impact our bodies. As we find ways to care for our bodily selves, with all its limitations and capabilities, the awareness of our physical needs grows—and so does our ability to attend to those needs. Some of our basic needs include eating, sleeping, intimate touch, and physical activity.

The kinds of questions I ask are open-ended:

- How is my body feeling right now—rested, nurtured, strong, tired, stressed, agitated, exhausted, etc.?
- What does my body need right now to be at its best?

- What is within my scope of control that I can start or stop doing?
- Who can help me figure this out?

Sometimes we can do some of this reflective work alone. Other times we need professional help.

2. Mind (beliefs, thoughts, emotions). What we allow our minds to engage in has a huge impact on our attitude and behaviour. Being intentional about our habits-of-mind can help us uncover what's helpful or unhelpful.

One way to determine whether something is helpful is to check in with ourselves and see how we feel when we think a certain way. What emotions surface? If it's helpful, we typically feel better, more peaceful, and more hopeful. If it's unhelpful, we tend to feel worse, unmotivated, overwhelmed, discouraged... maybe even stressed, worried, helpless, or hopeless. We may feel like a victim.

It's helpful to attune ourselves to what our inside voice says and listen to what we're listening to. Are we dwelling on something negative or figuring out a way to process it to make sense of it? Are we resisting and resenting a particular situation or learning to find ways to accept our reality? Are we looking at only the negative side or is there a modicum of good to see in the situation?

Looking at a crisis only through a lens of negativity keeps us stuck. Stuck emotionally, stuck in our old story.

Admittedly, negative thinking may be our first response, but as time passes, with love, support, care, and healing, along with faithfully cultivating margin, we can do the important and necessary work of gaining new perspectives. As we do this, we enter into a process of rebuilding and strengthening our resilience, which helps us find new ways to cope and embrace our lives.

If we're stuck, it might result in us having thoughts based in judgment, blame, resentment, unforgiveness, fantasy, and victim thinking. We may wonder, "If this hadn't happened, I'd probably be happy now." Repeatedly ruminating on negative thoughts can entrench our negative perceptions, keeping us stuck. This causes us to vent and ruminate, over and over.

Repeatedly venting isn't helpful because it tends to heighten our emotions, which can block our ability to be open and curious, or to change. It can also limit our ability to process our experiences and make meaning from them. When we vent, we bring up the same memories again and again, tying strong negative emotions to them, entrenching that negativity.

And be aware that the process of repeatedly recalling and dwelling on a memory, usually from a negative perspective, can alter its accuracy. Our memories change each time we recall them, massaging them with our assumptions and perceptions. So what we think we know happened may not even be accurate. These altered memories can become false stories we tell ourselves and others.

We must be careful about which stories we tell ourselves. Unbridled venting can keep us going in circles, allowing emotional automatic reactions to rule us. This inhibits our ability to cope or accept the sometimes difficult reality of our situations.

Understanding what's underneath our emotions and reactions is important. Processing and reframing them helps. Sometimes we do this on our own, but for many of us this process needs to be witnessed and coached in a safe place with a qualified professional.

Here are some examples of the open-ended questions I ask myself:

- What kinds of thoughts do I repeatedly have as I think about this situation?
- What do I think is true that may not be, and what kind of story do I tell myself about this?
- Does the way I think about a certain situation make me feel better or worse? Does the way I think make me move closer to people or pull back and want to isolate?
- What can I start doing to change what's within my scope of control?
- How do I move through this—learning, growing, and coping to function more effectively in life?
- Who can help me figure out how to do this?

It's not about taking on an attitude of toxic positivity or toxic negativity; it's about looking at our situation with hope-filled optimism. We don't dismiss the difficulties we face, nor the consequences with which we must learn to live.

Through this process, we can focus on a situation more holistically, helping us to better understand what we need in order to take care of ourselves along the way to healing. By choosing optimism with hope, over time and with practice, our thoughts and attitudes about an experience can change.

We must stop avoiding challenges and instead think about them as a part of life. These are opportunities to equip ourselves, rest, learn, doubt, trust, explore, understand, and make

We must stop avoiding challenges and instead think about them as a part of life.

sense of things. These are also chances to release attachments that may be keeping us stuck. We change and grow through this kind of healing process, helping us to live well in the journey.

There is no magic formula for learning to cope in adversity. We all need to figure it out for ourselves, because we are all different, with different backgrounds and different crises. Watching for the clues in our thoughts, words, body, and behaviour helps us determine when we might be experiencing a lack of margin.

My warning signs show up when I'm tired, stressed, or worried. When waves of grief are triggered or negative thinking creeps in, I tend to lose perspective and forget what I know to be true. This makes rest and sleep elusive, which perpetuates the cycle if I'm not diligent about monitoring my inner self. When I have a busy schedule, I sometimes put off my regular spiritual practices and tell myself I'll do them later. This is a warning sign that I'm relying on myself too much. When these signs show up, I often feel like I'm unable to bounce back as usual.

Thinking is the weak link in my soul care. My mind is regularly overactive, since I'm inquisitive, analytical, independent, and a problem solver. I often get myself into trouble by thinking too much, getting stuck down some unhelpful rabbit hole. As I monitor my own thinking processes and sift through what's unhelpful, I intentionally seek new, helpful thoughts.

One phrase I have incorporated this year is "Even so…" These words help me with acceptance, to live without answers to my questions. They help me live with the unknowns, pushing me into deeper levels of trust.

I've had cancer, surgery, and treatment, which has produced physical alterations in my looks and in the way I function. *Even so*, I am still good enough. I have much to be thankful for and I trust that God will use it for good. The promise of goodness is a gift I gratefully accept. I try to incorporate this into my life every day.

This phrase, "even so," helps me carry on and trust in God's bigger plans, because He knows more than I do. I deeply believe in the goodness of God. When I firmly believe that God is able to work all things for good, I feel free to take my eyes off myself and shift my focus from looking solely at the negative parts of my circumstances to things that bring life, hope, and joy.

Daily, I try to remember and cultivate habits to look forward with hope-filled optimism, anticipating the ways in which God will use my circumstances for good. This is good for Him, good for me, and good for others.

3. Spirit. The spirit is the deepest part of us, and it's the part that makes us fully alive. It's the part of us that seeks God, prays to God, longs for God—even when we aren't aware of it. We must listen to our deepest longings.

Here are some open-ended questions I ask myself when I assess the condition of my spirit:

- What are my thoughts regarding this situation?
- Where can I see God at work in this situation?
- What kind of longing or void do I sense within myself?
- How do I tend to fill this longing or void? What or who do I reach for to make myself feel better? What helps me, and what doesn't help?
- What does my spirit need in order for me to thrive?

• Does the way I think make me move closer to people or pull back and isolate from people? Do I move closer to God or further away from God?

Gaining awareness about why we choose to reach for a specific person, place, or thing can provide us with valuable information. Sometimes our deepest longings can only be filled spiritually even though we may attempt to fill ourselves with substitutions that may not be as life-giving. In fact, they could even be bad for us.

During these trying times, it's important to remain open to cultivating spiritual growth. This requires being intentional about our inner world and regularly ridding ourselves of the weeds which choke out our spiritual health. Instead we must feed ourselves with life-giving nutrients and light that can pour new life into us along the way.

We must identify helpful practices in our lives that are sustainable. Many people practice spiritual disciplines like meditation, silence, reading, prayer, walking, journalling, being in community, being creative, etc. All the while, we must also allow ourselves to acknowledge, attend to, and release sadness, sorrow, anger, and challenges that emerge; we must not minimize or dismiss them.

Taking a holistic approach to soul care will lead us into deeper faith and abiding hope. Faith and hope will help us to develop more wholeness along the way. After all, we were designed to be whole.

Cultivating Regular Rhythms
Soul care requires us to follow regular rhythms. Each of us needs to figure out what works best, whether it be daily practices that last five to twenty minutes, or weekly practices. Some of us may even benefit from taking a full retreat day from time to time to escape the hustle and bustle of life. No matter what amount of time we dedicate to this, it will benefit us and we will grow.

When I faithfully practice daily rhythms of soul care, I ask myself reflective questions. I need to take the necessary time to consider and answer them, not just skim over them. Meditating on such reflective questions makes me think about the kind of person I feel called to be, the kind of person I want to be known for.

On days when emotional struggles return—like when I'm triggered by a new spot or lump, experience strong muscle spasms, or undergo a minor surgical procedure—I need a reminder that spots come as we age, and some pain comes with healing. These aren't always signs of danger. And I must remember that medical procedures are sometimes necessary. When undertaken for good reasons, they help to maintain my health and well-being.

Practicing my favourite soul care disciplines helps me return to a place of equilibrium and peace without minimizing or dismissing the current difficulty. We need to integrate our losses and enter life with health and purpose instead of getting stuck in the past or in fear. Integrating our losses is about accepting our reality, dealing with it, and allow us to change into new and better versions of ourselves. And it includes cultivating a heart of gratitude for what we had in the past and may no longer have today. We also trust in a good future, anticipating with hope what is to come.

The challenge is in choosing to live well every day, even when there are difficult days to face.

As I've already said, I have come to learn that the challenge with having been given a diagnosis of cancer is not in medical details. The challenge is in choosing to live well every day, even when there are difficult days to face.

Let's embrace life, embrace hope, and embrace the best version of ourselves in the midst of the crisis. Let's choose to embrace life-giving thoughts, life-giving emotions, life-giving activities, and life-giving relationships.

HIGHLIGHTS

What if we can become better equipped so we can become more resilient? Maybe we can become the best version of ourselves and be more real along the way, which will help us choose to live well in the next part of our story.

Reflections

Consider What Keeps Us Stuck

- Repeatedly venting isn't helpful because it tends to heighten our emotions, which can block our ability to be open, curious, or change. It limits our ability to process well and make meaning from our experiences.

Consider What Brings Life

- Body, mind, and spirit are all part of God's original design of humanity. We were originally designed to be whole.
- Soul care helps us become more resilient in responding to the necessary changes we face, especially when we attend to ourselves as whole people—body, mind, and spirit.

Personal Reflection

- Think of one area of your life right now in which you could use some margin. If you had margin in this area, what would be different for you?
- What is one soul care activity that could bring life if you practice it? See Appendix A for some ideas.
- What is one way in which you could practice using an "even so" statement in your life?

Chapter Eight

ENDURING HOPE

Hope is the inevitable product of a life that chooses to love.[30]

—Thich Truong

NOT ONLY DOES THE word hope hold different meanings in different contexts, but it elicits different responses from us depending on our expectations about what hope promises.

For example, we might express hope for the weather to change or hope that a friend will feel better. This kind of hope describes a longing, preference, or understanding that our expressed desire might not be fulfilled.

Then there's the kind of hope for the future that says, "I hope I'll get a dog for my birthday" or "I hope I'll be chosen for an interview." This kind of hope keeps us daydreaming about what it will be like should our hopes come true. This hope is more compelling than the first example. It's tied up with more uncertainty because we can't predict the outcome. We feel a greater degree of disappointment if the hope isn't realized.

Then there's the kind of hope, which is still deeper and greater, that knows with absolute certainty that something will come to pass because of the character of the One who gives it. When we know the giver—their character, motive, promise, and purpose—we possess an assuredness that causes us to trust the promise will come to pass. It's a hope filled with expectancy.

John Piper defines biblical hope this way: "a confident expectation and desire for something good in the future."[31] When we know that God is good, that His character never changes, and that He loves us, wants good for us, and His promises are always true and never fail, we develop confidence in Him. This gives us the strength and perseverance to live with hope-filled anticipation for what is to come.

God is the only one who knows the bigger purpose behind what happens around us. Since we see only in part, there will always be mystery. When we can find it in our hearts to trust God's Word, including His work, plans, and promise that He will bring good out of every situation, we are filled with hopeful anticipation—even when it's difficult to see goodness.

For me, this type of enduring hope comes with the certainty of an abundant life, to be lived right now despite our circumstances. It brings healing and wholeness and looks forward with expectant, confident anticipation of what God will do. It's hope filled with faith and trust in the promise of eternal life when we die.

This hope is available to anyone who chooses to have faith in, believe in, and trust in God's promises. With this hope present deep inside us, our heart shifts subtly and we go from being consumers of the world to stewards of it, from being self-focused to other-focused, from being selfish to generous, from being resentful to thankful, from striving to becoming, from taking to giving, from resenting to forgiving. We become more the kind of person we were originally designed to be.

When tragedy strikes, we can embrace an enduring hope through which we learn to loosen our grip on our preferred expectations and learn to see and welcome things differently—in ways that brings wholeness, insight, growth, and new perspectives.

Instead of seeing others, the world, material things, or God as resources available solely to meet our own expectations to make us happy, a divine shift emerges. With time our eyes and hearts open to see the gifts that have been sitting before us all along. Each person or thing before us is a gift, a treasure to be cherished. The difficult times we experience become opportunities to release that which hinders, to learn and grow. In these times, our perspectives are transformed. Previously ordinary moments, such as experiencing the beauty of nature or loving our friends and family, become precious.

When we receive these gifts with praise and gratitude, we move out of the centre of the universe and let God take His rightful place as we take ours.

Uncovering Hope

Although I came to see that the challenge of getting through a crisis like cancer isn't about receiving the diagnosis and recovery but in choosing to live well regardless, I didn't always think that way. Early on, I struggled with wanting to go back to "normal." My goal was to get better and then live the same way I had before the diagnosis.

But that would have been impossible.

My sole focus was on physical restoration. Unwittingly I had embraced a very narrow definition of health, healing, and wholeness.

Not long ago, a friend showed me a paragraph written by author John Swinton. In *Finding Jesus in the Storm*, Swinton writes about the meaning of health:

> Scripture has no equivalent term for biomedical understandings of health that equates health with the absence of illness. The closest term is the Hebrew term *shalom*, which has a core meaning of righteousness, holiness, right relationship with God. From this perspective, to be healthy is to be in right relationship with God regardless of one's physical or psychological state. One can be the world's fittest athlete, the world's richest, most hedonistic individual, or the most psychologically stable person on the planet and still be deeply unhealthy. Health in this perspective is not a medical or a psychological concept but primarily a relational and theological concept. Health is not the absence of anything; it's the presence of God.[32]

We were originally designed for wholeness. When we invite God into our lives, He guides the process of integrating our mind, body, and spirit in surprising ways. This may not mean that we are cured from our disease or have a problem-free life, but we can still be whole—we see glimpses of wholeness here on the earth and will see it even more completely in heaven.

Furthermore, when we seek wholeness, we can find hope, joy, and strength along the way because God is with us. Because God is good, we can trust the eternal outcomes He promises.

For me, this indicates that the way we live is critical, no matter what we face. The presence of hope we all long for, especially when we experience suffering, is available to us.

Welcoming Hope

Hope can be cultivated through nurturing our spiritual growth. It's a journey of discovery, full of mystery and courage. Faith is its foundation.

Faith, of course, is the belief that we need something other than ourselves to survive and thrive instead of navigating life solely on our own. For many, it can lead us on a gradual spiritual awakening. Others may seek a clearer vision of God or renew their faith commitment while learning more about His purposes and ways.

Hope can be seen and defined in different ways. It can be defined as the action of having confidence in or trust in something, or it can be something for which we have a desire or wish.[33]

Hope is usually tied into whatever or whomever we put our faith. We tend to reach for something or someone when we lack hope. If our hope is in ourselves, we may attempt to get through in our own efforts. If our hope is in having things, we may try to gain more possessions. If our hope is in money, we may seek opportunities to accumulate money. If our hope is in being important, we may try to align ourselves with important people or vie to be the centre of attention.

If our hope is in God, we put our trust in Him.

In my faith tradition, we express our hope in God because of who He is—His nature, character, and promises. For me, learning more about God's character and purposes has led me to a place of greater trust and hopefulness in my own walk through cancer. It has helped me understand what true hope looks like and redefine what wholeness and healing is on the earth and in heaven.

Life involves transformation, for we become all that we were intended to be—whole. We can only do this when we have a full assurance of who God is.

There was a time, decades ago, when I just listened to historical opinion, misunderstandings, or inaccurate theologies about the nature of God. Yet when I finally did my own research and due diligence, I came to understand God's goodness and His desire for good for us.

Over the last thirty years, and especially in the last two years, my awareness of God's character has grown. I have become better able to accept His promises, purposes, and ways regardless of my circumstances, regardless of the mystery. It's an awareness through which, with necessary and regular reminders, I can trust God because I know that good will come out of the bad. I know that my circumstances right now aren't the end of my story.

I have never attributed blame to God for my circumstances. Why? Because sometimes bad stuff just happens. Evil exists in this world. Mankind has historically made poor decisions that have affected previous generations. This has been true since the beginning of time. I've made my own fair share of poor decisions. And sometimes we just don't have all the answers.

What helps me most is hanging on to God's promises:

- God is good.
- God loves us. We are God's beloved.
- God wants good for us, and He'll work all things for good.
- God brings shalom, true healing, and wholeness.
- God has plans for us and wants us to have hope.
- He is always with us.
- He transforms us more into the image He wants for us.
- He promises to redeem the world.

And best of all, when it's time for our lives in this world to come to an end, He gives us everlasting life. We will finally be fully whole and restored—body, soul, and spirit—the way we were originally intended to be. I can be thankful for these promises, thankful for the peace, comfort, and joy I receive despite setbacks.

As I continue in my adventure, I am committed to actively doing my part as a finite human still learning how to welcome wholeness in safe community while I put my faith, hope, and trust in God, for He will do His part according to His promises.

Joy, a Byproduct of Enduring Hope

One outcome that continues to surprise me is experiencing joy when I embrace this kind of enduring hope.

Writer Ronne Rock recently posted an eloquent reflection on joy that goes like this:

> I've been pondering joy as I consider the description of this amazing fruit scripture says is born from God's own presence in our lives—a fruit described as unconditional love, joy, peace, patience, kindheartedness, goodness, faithfulness, gentleness, and self-control. If love is at the very core of the fruit, then I think joy might be its pith. I know. Pith conjures up thoughts of the spongy white in-between bitterness hiding just under the skin of an orange or lemon. And to be honest, joy is perhaps a bit bittersweet in its presence.
>
> But as I reflect on the scripture, "The joy of the Lord is my strength," the purpose of pith comes into view. It is essential for the very life of the fruit, moving and storing nutrients in each cell. And the pith keeps the plant alive as it grows. Joy is God's strength embodied in us, not a thing to be acquired or chased or grasped. It is God's own character, His personality woven into the fiber of us. And it is His strength that keeps us moving. Joy is the whisper that hope is always near, that redemption is a possibility, that there is still good to be tasted.

Joy moves through the days when grief changes the composition of the air we breathe, or when frustration litters our path with stones, or when weariness threatens to wilt our souls. Joy is not daunted by fear or destroyed by a season of wondering or wandering. Joy is the strength that allows us to smile even though there are storms raging around us and within us as we dig our hands into the soil of the days to cultivate a life that is life-giving.[34]

I love her analogy of joy, because it grows from an enduring hope based on the character of God, not our circumstances, and gives us new ways of understanding joy. We can see glimpses of it even in times of suffering as we keep our eyes focused on the One who brings true joy and strength to persevere in times of suffering.

Hope in Community

As I look back and contemplate the ways in which I saw and experienced hope in and through my own cancer journey, I see God's fingerprints all over it, forging even more thankfulness and hope deep in my heart. This has led me to extend the parameters of how we can receive hope. This is the kind of hope that connects us to one another, relationally.

Embracing a tangible hope helps us to know that we aren't alone, that we are cared for by others. Such a hope brings sojourners into our lives to walk alongside us for a time. These sojourners help us persevere in the everyday moments when we struggle, bringing us words of hope and encouragement, helping us to keep our focus on that which brings life and wholeness.

I still experience hope in the ongoing, loving encouragement and acceptance I receive from my cherished husband. I experience hope through the loving attention and check-ins that come from my precious children and older siblings. I experience hope through the faithful prayers, quiet conversations, and adventures I enjoy with my valued friends. I experience hope through interactions with my surgeon, who makes me laugh at each appointment. I experience hope with the many other doctors. One even put my name and a happy face on a sticky note on her computer, saying that she sent me "good thoughts" each time she saw the happy face reminder. All these people provide excellent ongoing care for me and continually make deposits of hope that I feel deep in my heart.

I experienced that kind of hope through the ICU nurse as she spoke words of encouragement only hours after my surgery. I experienced that hope through caring interactions with the hospital staff who pushed me to persevere. And I felt it from the surgeons, residents, interns, nurses, nutritionists, occupational therapists, physiotherapists, speech therapists, respiratory therapists, the oncologist, and radiology technicians who worked on my case. They are all amazing.

It's as though each of these individuals have stood in the gap for me, holding me up on difficult days, helping me to keep my focus while encouraging me to take the next step. To me, this is a foretaste of God's goodness and promise of wholeness—a little bit of heaven while still on the earth. God uses people to bring hope and perseverance amidst challenges. We are made for community, designed to care for one another, since we are made in God's image.

I've even experienced hope through the many images, thoughts, memories, and insights I have received over these last two years. I often wonder if they too are gentle brush strokes of gold from God, as they bubble up into my awareness. I accept each one of them with gratitude.

Yet having hope doesn't mean we won't face difficulties, suffer, or become exhausted or discouraged. It does, however, mean that we'll be infused with the courage, wholeness, and strength to persevere, no matter how small the steps we take. It's a type of hope that doesn't despair. Sometimes this kind of hope is hard to see, but it will come, because as we place our full assurance in God's character, His promises, and in our ultimate future, this is the gift we receive. Because He is a God of restoration, He can restore our hope. It's His promise to restore us and make us whole.

This is the hope we can experience on the earth while we're alive. But in the end, when our time here is done, there is also hope available to us in the form of experiencing eternal life in heaven. And when we die, we can have hope filled with assurance in the gift of eternal life—a gift that is good because God is good.

Bringing Hope to Others

My period of recovery from cancer was a cherished yet poignant time for me to text and pray for a dear friend who subsequently lost her decade-long battle with cancer.

We chuckled as we reminisced about a ski date we once went on, having snuck off for a day to go downhill skiing in the Rocky Mountains. With each passing hour, we had gotten braver, trying more challenging runs. My friend, an avid snowboarder, had wanted to introduce me to moguls—little piles of snow hills interspersed along a ski run usually reserved for skilled skiers. She went first, slicing back and forth, as though she were simply icing a cake. She made it look easy and my own confidence soared as she seamlessly made it to the bottom of the trail.

That doesn't look too bad, I thought. *I can do this!*

Looking up she waved—it was my turn. Although I had skied for most of my life, I had never been brave enough to try moguls.

Blindly inspired by my friend's exceptional skill, I set out.

Reaching the first mogul, I prepared myself to be propelled slightly into the air. I bent my knees, stuck out my butt, and balanced my body evenly over the skis—or so I thought. Suddenly my feet shot out from under me and I flew up into the air. It felt like slow motion as my body floated higher and higher. My skis moved into a ninety-degree position and my crouched body stretched into a face-up, spreadeagle pose.

Then gravity kicked in. I fell to the ground with a sickening thud, landing on my back. My helmet-less head flung backward, thwacking down onto the packed snow. With the wind knocked out of me, I lay still for a moment before moving various body parts to ensure nothing was broken.

Nothing appeared broken—the rib I had unwittingly popped out of place, however, made it painful to move and breathe.

Laughter soon erupted as I imagined the sight of me soaring like an upside-down eagle.

My friend scooted up the hill sideways with a concerned look on her face. She checked on me before we both slowly skied down to the ski lodge to rest and recover. Filled with warm hot chocolate, within the hour my friend convinced me to do one last *easy* run so I would have a good final memory of our day.

Reminiscing about the shenanigans we experienced together brought enjoyment and connection, providing a bit of distraction and relief.

As fellow cancer patients, we felt less alone because we understood each other's experiences about the unexpected muscle spasms and pain, not to mention thinking about the food we had to eat to maintain weight and blood counts. We even shared tips on recipes. It seemed comfortable to speak authentically about our shared reality without someone feeling sorry for us, or labelling us as a condition. We were more than just cancer patients.

And of course the reality is that we'll all die someday. I think many forget this simple fact of life until it's their turn.

It was a bittersweet time. She inspired me with much courage and hope, yet I was also saddened that such a beautiful, kind-hearted woman would leave her family and friends so early in life.

Only after she was gone did I come to learn that I was one of the few women with whom she had connected through the last few months of her life. This is an honour I will always cherish. And it's a valuable lesson for me to never, ever assume I have nothing to offer. It's not true that I can't offer help just because I don't know what to say. I can encourage another person even through a simple call, prayer, text, or meal.

Since my diagnosis, I've been given many other opportunities to encourage people newly diagnosed with cancer—some with oral cancer like me. I don't necessarily feel equipped and I don't always know what to say, but I am reminded of how encouraged I was with the hope-filled words from those who sojourned with me. I consider it a privilege to reciprocate when I can.

After offering encouragement to others, I noticed to my surprise that I had more energy, motivation, and vitality in my own life. I also realized that although I wasn't the same as I had been before the diagnosis, I could still accomplish much despite my limitations. These opportunities of giving back gave me courage, confidence, much-needed purpose, and greater hope to persevere and welcome new wholeness.

Serving others in need normalizes our own needs when they arise. Suffering is a universal experience; no one escapes it. It cultivates compassion and love for one another. It's a unifying experience that helps us to realize no one is immune from crisis.

Helping others is never a replacement for dealing with our own suffering, but it can become an outworking of compassion for our fellow man.

Suffering is a universal experience...

Most beneficially of all, it affirms that we need each other. We are made for community—a healthy environment of love that gives us an opportunity to sojourn with, encourage, and become a witness to others who are suffering. This is a healing, life-giving, intimate gift of love, one to another.

God Is a Source of Hope

Amidst the tears and suffering I have experienced, several things have brought me hope. First is a deep and abiding trust in a God who gives promises and keeps His promises.

I remind myself that leaning on Him doesn't mean bad things won't happen to me. It doesn't mean we won't suffer. And it doesn't mean all our dreams will be magically fulfilled.

However, it does mean that we're responsible for doing our part in embracing wholeness as active participants in life and our world while trusting God will do His. It does mean that God is with us and for us, even if we sometimes don't sense it. He is a God who draws close to us as we draw close to Him. He's a God who can use anything for good.

Faith helps us to gain greater insight. Faith doesn't alienate; it brings things together. Faith doesn't discount modern medicine and skilled surgeons, research, or statistics. It doesn't discount the benefits of psychologists, physiotherapists, and other professional supports we may need along the way. These are all good gifts created by God as a blessing to help us, because whatever is good comes from God.

Faith, Hope, and Love

Faith and hope are linked. We can't have faith without hope, and we can't have hope without faith. Embodying faith means trusting that God is good and that He is who He says He is. This is the hope we receive despite our circumstances, allowing us to continue to move forward—hope on earth, and hope in heaven.

Faith and hope are linked to love—God's love for us. He is love and wants what's best for us. He doesn't want us to suffer, and this is shown by His redemptive plan for each one of us in Jesus Christ's sacrifice and the inheritance given to those who choose to receive it.

By working through our own crises and disappointments through a lens of faith, hope, and love, we change the ending of our own story, and this leads us to become more of who God created us to be—body, soul, and spirit. Enduring hope arrives as we choose to live well, not dependent upon our circumstances but upon God.

It's my desire that sharing my story and the insights I've been learning along the way might inspire you to embrace life and embrace hope in new and life-giving ways. And as you seek enduring hope, may you also find shalom.

HIGHLIGHTS

Hope is the certainty of being able to experience an abundant life now despite our circumstances. Hope is looking forward with confident anticipation of what God will do. Hope is having faith and trust in the promise of eternal life when we die.

Reflections

Consider What Keeps Us Stuck

- Become more aware of what we're thinking, where we place our faith and hope, and what brings life and what doesn't.

Consider What Brings Life

- Practice the art of remembering that which we tend to forget—all that brings goodness and life to our hearts.

Personal Reflection

- What is one thing that helps you find joy?
- What does the pith represent in your own life?
- What one life-giving experience can you invite into your life that cultivates wholeness?
- What one life-giving experience are you resisting that could help you cultivate wholeness?

SOUL CARE PRACTICES

Finally, brothers and sisters, whatever is true, whatever is noble, whatever is right, whatever is pure, whatever is lovely, whatever is admirable— if anything is excellent or praiseworthy—think about such things. Whatever you have learned or received or heard from me, or seen in me—put it into practice. And the God of peace will be with you. (Philippians 4:8–9)

INTENTIONALLY ATTENDING TO OURSELVES as a whole person—body, mind, and spirit—is soul care. Soul care speaks to the many ways in which we can cultivate a simpler, gentler way of life, doing what is good for us while making investments in our overall health and daily lives.

Caring for our soul is like strengthening muscle. Our muscles strengthen when we make intentional, repeated, slow, careful movement in both directions—up and down. Before I enrolled in a fitness class for cancer patients, I thought that strengthening a muscle meant lifting bigger and heavier weights. But it's actually in the slow, deliberate lengthening and release of the muscle.

The same is true of our souls. When we release what is unhelpful and bring in what is helpful, we strengthen our souls—our resilience. Through this act of release, we make room for good to grow in us. This builds inner strength.

Soul care, like building and strengthening a muscle, isn't something to be rushed. We don't start with the big stuff, the heavy weights. We start with small ones. We become intentional about our form, movement, and speed. We repeat the exercise regularly until we see results. We isolate different muscle groups to concentrate our efforts on the areas that need attention. We set goals, schedule time to exercise, and build in time to rest and recover. And as we are diligent and become stronger, our muscles become better able to sustain us, keep us balanced, and help us recover in the face of a fall.

By developing, exploring, and practicing regular rhythms of soul care we learn what is best to release, and what helps create room for us to be filled with faith, insight, hope, and strength. This process helps us find ways to accept our circumstances, deal with the emotional turmoil, and look to our future with new perspectives despite our loss. When future challenges or crises happen, these practices will form a firm foundation.

Soul care activities will help us enter more deeply into becoming more real and whole, walking through life with hope. We all need hope.

Practicing Soul Care

Soul care requires quiet uninterrupted time to attend to what's going on inside us. When I had younger children, I set up a small table in our bedroom and covered it with a pretty tablecloth. On the table I placed a candle, a few favourite books, and a journal to use during my quiet times. This simple start acted as a visual reminder to take time for soul care, which I needed as a busy part-time professional and full-time mother.

Once our daughters married and left home, I converted one of their bedrooms into a small art studio that now doubles as a quiet room. This is where I keep my artwork, music, books, journals, and watercolour art supplies. This is my sacred space—a quiet place where interruptions don't occur. If the door is closed, nothing and no one interrupts me. It's also where I acknowledge my deep needs for healing, wholeness, and God.

This appendix contains a few of my favourite soul care activities and the spiritual disciplines that have proven useful over many decades. Time and practical experience have helped me identify which ones are most effective based on who I am and how I'm wired. They have been instrumental in reminding me of the need to set aside time to be alone with God, and with myself, to learn what's getting in the way of becoming whole—body, soul, and spirit.

When I do, I'm a better me. These tools have been invaluable in terms of helping me find ways to share my heart with God and learn how to listen to His still, quiet voice in my life. And they have helped me find new ways to make meaning from some of the crossroads I've experienced in my life.

Not only can soul care practices help us find ways to make sense of our lives, but they also have the potential to help us become open to God's transformation, drawing us deeper into the understanding and practicing of our faith. They help us carve out time to allow God to transform us, both in the best of times and the worst. These disciplines cultivate a welcoming stance in which we become more open to the change that comes only through spending quality time with God as we seek His wisdom, insight, truth, and hope.

Jesus modelled for us what a whole life is intended to look like. It's a life filled with preparation, spiritual growth, and love—even suffering. It's being intimately connected to God and to others. In studying His life, I have come to learn that He showed us how important it is, despite the busy demands of life, to spend time in solitude to be with God.

Jesus lived in community alongside others and His life was filled with action based in love, compassion, and service for others. He modelled a life filled with purpose and mission—one of sacrifice, suffering, forgiveness, and redemption.

Spending time with God transforms our motives and character, giving us time to uncover that which holds us back from healing, growth, and wholeness. Soul care and spiritual disciplines are designed to deepen our faith and draw us closer to God.

As outlined in Chapter Seven, my soul care activities have four key components: receiving in, reaching up, reflecting and releasing, and reaching out.

After decades of practice, I have accumulated different activities from which to draw for each of these stages. Depending on the day and time available, I'll pick and choose what fits best for the moment.

Below is a list of the kinds of activities I undertake for my own soul care. For a few of my favourites, I'll provide a brief example and a list of my helpful reading resources.

In the beginning, I started with just one activity, practiced it, and then as I saw value in it I became more committed. Bit by bit, I added more activities to help me continue growing. I don't do every activity every single day. Sometimes it's just one or two.

Receiving in activities:
- Breath prayer.
- Deep breathing and muscle relaxation.
- Reading Scripture and following my daily prayer guide.

Reaching up activities:
- Reading a helpful book on a topic I'm researching.
- Time for quiet reflection.
- Prayer.

Reflecting and releasing activities:
- Practice of quiet solitude and silence.
- Being mindful and present in the here and now, acutely aware of the thoughts cluttering my mind.
- Acknowledging my needs and desires.
- Reflecting (motives, meaning, purposes, etc.).
- Cultivating a sense of humour.
- Offering forgiveness to myself and others.
- Journalling my reflections.
- Creative activity (I'm a watercolour artist, spending many afternoons painting while listening to music, especially when homebound in the winter months).
- Examen prayer.

Reaching out activities:
- Taking daily walks with my husband and dog.
- Having fun—kayaking, camping (yes, in a tent), playing games, walking, or sharing meals with friends.

- Engaging in regular exercise that includes cardio, strengthening, challenges, and fun.
- Meeting new people by taking classes, joining groups, building community, etc.
- During the fall and winter, I get together every week or two with friends while reading a book on personal or spiritual growth and reflect upon what we are learning together.
- Engaging in meaningful connection with beloved family members and friends.
- Participating in a monthly book club.
- Keeping my eyes open and intentionally offering words of encouragement to those facing crises.
- Volunteering in meaningful ways that are doable and suitable given my circumstances.

I'm considering adding another "R" to my list: *rejoicing*. This is something I'm learning to cultivate and integrate with deep thankfulness. It's similar to gratitude, but deeper because it includes thoughtful articulation about the reasons we are grateful, with an emphasis on the physical, emotional, and spiritual impact rejoicing has on us. I also focus on the source of rejoicing. This includes remembering and calling up that warm, fuzzy feeling we get when we're pleasantly surprised by an unexpected blessing—maybe because it comes from God since He is the source of all good things.

My goal is to continue cultivating these practices to help them become a more deeply ingrained way of life wherein I can embrace more of what brings peace, wholeness, goodness, and life to me and those around me. With faithful practice I hope it will bring me to a place where I can have closeness with others and a deeper walk with God— one that continues to transform the real me and my character while also deepening my faith, hope, and joy as I become more whole each day.

My Favourite Soul Care Activities

Breath prayers. Sometimes when I can't do anything else but breathe, I take a short scripture or prayer to recite, using it to breathe deeply. I need regular reminders that God is the one who gives us breath—and without breath, we would not have life.

A breath prayer is a great way to pray to God when our own words feel insufficient or are difficult to articulate. It's a time to remind ourselves who God is and Whose we are. It also creates space in our hearts, expands our breath, reduces stress, helps us relax, and brings more oxygen into our body.

When challenges come my way, I often use this sentence from John 14:27 as a slow, deep breath prayer: *"Peace I leave with you; my peace I give you..."* I split it into two breaths—an in-breath and an out-breath, each for a count of four. I breathe slowly with a selection of word combinations that fit... 1–2–3–4, 1–2–3–4... followed by a pause, then 1–2–3–4... Then I repeat the sequence until I sense deep inner calm and peace in my heart.

There are many ways to breathe; this is just one that works for me. It helped me when I couldn't breathe, when I was undergoing radiation, when I get bad news, when I have trouble sleeping, or when I awaken in the middle of the night. It helps me prepare my heart for quiet times.

Mindful presence. A good number of us allow our minds to run amok, and in the process we tend to react to difficult situations instead of responding in a more thoughtful way. How do we know which thoughts are helpful and which aren't?

Thoughts that make me feel bad, angry, impatient, frustrated, depressed, jealous, resentful, or full of self-pity distance me from God and the person I want to be known for. These thoughts go on my *unhelpful* list. Thoughts that lead me to feel good, peaceful, patient, compassionate, content, confident, and full of joy draw me closer to God and the person I want to be. They go on my *helpful* list.

It's a good versus bad list, and some spiritual directors call it *consolation* (that which draws us close to God) versus *desolation* (that which draws us away from God). Some folks may name them truth versus lies, helpful versus unhelpful.

Our thoughts can influence our behaviours and take us in a specific direction. Toward or away from people, toward or away from God. We must be careful about what we allow ourselves to think and be aware of what we tell ourselves in times of suffering and loss. We can easily become fixated on our circumstances and overly influenced by pain and its associated thoughts and assumptions, which may not necessarily be true.

A common thought when something bad happens to us is "I'm the only one." Or we may believe, "There's something wrong with me" or "I'm being punished" or "It's my own fault; I deserve this." In many cases, these thoughts aren't true.

In the same manner that taking a wrong turn can make us lose time down the road, unhelpful thinking and believing lies can take us down a path we were never intended to travel. In doing so, we waste critical energy, taking up important space that clutters the mind, inhibiting our ability to see truth clearly or consider alternative ways of thinking and being.

There are many good books, programs, therapists, psychologists, spiritual directors, and ministers that can help uncover unhelpful ways of thinking. I'll not go into them here, but I encourage you to research the subject to see if new learning could benefit you as it did me.

It can be helpful to cultivate a way to notice what we're thinking and how our body physically responds to a situation. This helps us become aware of our unhelpful thoughts and reactions. We don't have to wait for a crisis to learn how to do this.

Many mindful activities are available to help us create space and allow our emotional resilience to grow and develop, calming our racing thoughts and creating enough margin for us to find new ways to think and be in this world.

The practice of being present is an excellent exercise. When we are present to ourselves, we become more aware of our thoughts and bodily sensations, and we may even notice things around us we never noticed before. As we learn to do this, we can become more aware of, and present with, others and God instead of being distracted.

When I first learned about this idea of being present, decades ago, I evaluated where my thoughts went. I quickly realized that I spent more time thinking about the future than anything else. I smugly called it being proactive and thought it was a good skill to have. I also spent some time thinking about the past and allowed myself to dwell on what I could have done differently. I justified it as helping me to continuously improve myself because I wanted things in my life to get better. But really I was participating in the art of avoiding the present, instead dwelling on a past that couldn't be changed and a future that couldn't be controlled. Placing too much focus on an unknown future can create anxiety; too much focus on an unchangeable past can create discouragement or second-guessing.

Future, past, fantasy. We all do it. The big question is how much we do it and how much of our time is spent in all those other places instead of in the present—the here and now.

I would ask myself two important questions. When I spend copious amounts of time in the past and future, what am I missing now in the present? And what would be a more healthy, balanced, or acceptable goal for me to work toward?

Once I figured out where my mind and thoughts ventured, I made a commitment to try being more present to myself and to others. Over the next few months, I set out to break my tendencies to worry about the future and dwell on the past.

With this goal in mind, I set a timer to chime every hour, no matter where I was, and I'd ask myself, *Where am I?* Then I would consider the location of my thoughts—past, present, future, or fantasy—and engage in a short grounding exercise. I'd look around and ask questions that engaged my senses, bringing me back to the present: *What do I see? What can I touch? What can I hear? What can I smell? What can I taste?*

It took a while, but eventually, with persistence, I was able to practice being present with greater ease.

I recall the exact moment when I first noticed I became fully present without distraction. I stood at the kitchen sink slowly peeling a carrot for supper. Looking down at my hands, I listened to the slice of the blade running along the carrot as it slowly stripped off the thin outer layer. I watched the peel bend and twist into the sink and smelled the aroma of fresh carrot as juice sprayed backward, depositing a few cold drops onto my hand.

My mind was focused on preparing the dish. I wasn't thinking about anything else. I had not mentally exited the room by visiting the past, present, or future. I wasn't daydreaming. I was right there, in the present, preparing supper—without any of the distractions that typically took my mind elsewhere.

Surprisingly, I enjoyed every moment of being present—the smell and feel of the carrot. It was a moment I'll never forget.

Since then, I regularly practice the art of being present, and in the process I've come to notice more details around me that I never saw before. I now pick up on all sorts of human facial cues many others might miss. I'm more self-aware of my inner stirrings, longings, and needs and have gotten better at taking the necessary time to attend to them in my self-care and soul care.

My self-awareness and other-awareness have definitely increased from this practice and I am a more authentic *me*.

Once we can be present to ourselves, we are better able to give that gift of presence to others—a very healing gift for them to experience.

Have you ever had someone give you the gift of being present? Present in your story, in your pain, and in your journey? This isn't about giving advice or being an expert or know-it-all. It's just about being totally present in a way that allows you to feel heard or understood. It's life-giving.

These kinds of people are the ones who provide a safe place to explore, remaining silent but also present and attentive, always with gentle and accepting eye contact, listening to the story, and asking important questions. They're often able to offer thoughtful insights and give encouragement when asked.

Often they just listen. And when they speak, their words are few but deeply impactful.

Being present to another is a special gift of hope for someone in crisis, someone who needs to be heard and valued.

Sense of humour. One surprising thing I noticed early on is that I find myself laughing a lot more. I'm better able to find humour even in the challenges and limitations of this new version of myself.

I recall the pleasure I found one day in the simple activity of trying to communicate while in the hospital. I was downloading a simple phone app that would convert text to voice, allowing me to communicate electronically with my nurses. As I watched everyone's response to the funny little computerized voice, I realized that they were all having fun too. This experience gave me much-needed joy in the first few difficult days of my ordeal. It was a necessary distraction from the challenge of recovering from surgery.

Later, I was readmitted to the hospital with a neck infection, although this time I was classified as an "independent" patient. At first I didn't realize the freedom this label brought with it. When I asked the nurses to send someone to get a bag of clothes and books from my husband at the hospital's front entrance, they suggested that I go get it myself!

What? Had I been given a get-out-of-jail-free card? Excitedly I brushed my hair, then carefully, one-handedly put on my mascara and put on my bra. I needed to look as good as I could for my husband, especially if I was going to be walking around the hospital. I struggled a bit with the logistics of putting on the bra, since I still had one arm lightly bandaged while the other was connected to an IV.

A nice nurse who happened by facilitated my quick disconnect from the machine and helped me dress. I decided to slip on a hospital housecoat to mitigate the potential breezes through the gaping opening in the back of the gown.

Once dressed, the nurse hooked me back up to the IV and unplugged it from the wall. With that, I put on my face mask and shoes, grabbed the IV pole, and set out to meet my husband.

In my excitement, I took the wrong elevator down—the one orderlies used to transport patients—and got hopelessly lost. I had difficulty communicating with people I met along the corridor and received many confused looks and "Pardons." My tongue was tired from slowly enunciating through the mask, which made my speech even more garbled than normal.

After the third set of directions, I finally made it to the front door.

I saw my husband standing patiently by the revolving doors, masked, bundled in a winter coat, and carrying a small bag of items to help make my second hospital stay more comfortable. He opened his arms, embraced me, and snuggled me in close. My face nuzzled safely into the crook of his soft, warm neck while my tears dripped onto his coat. It had only been twenty-four hours, yet it still seemed cruel that I once again couldn't have any visitors.

We stood there unashamedly with our arms wrapped around each other while other masked people quietly moved past us.

Many hours later, I decided it was time to crawl back into bed and read.

Like most women with years of practice, I can undo my bra under my clothes with one hand, even with an IV in my arm. I reached inside the housecoat, into the opening, and unsnapped the hooks, slipping one arm out and then trying to pull the other arm through the bra and down the arm sleeve simultaneously. What was usually a seamless, confident movement quickly became a challenge.

I realized there was absolutely no place for my bra to go but to slip off my arm and dangle like a giant Halloween costume, reminding me of oversized fairy wings flapping freely from the IV tube still attached to the needle in my arm. I forgot that the nurse had unhooked me in the morning.

Now what was I going to do? Sinking down on the edge of my bed, it occurred to me that I couldn't slip the bra over my head. I couldn't take it off, and I certainly couldn't put it back on! There would be no hiding this one...

I considered leaving it hanging and fixing it in the morning, but if I did that I wouldn't be able to take off the housecoat either.

Maybe I'll leave the coat on all night, I thought. *It'll keep me warm. But then I might get too hot in these old hospital rooms.*

Gazing down at the dangling bra, I wondered whether I should ask for help.

Memories and images flashed through my head from the last time I had seen bras hanging from places they were not meant to hang. Late one fall evening, under the cover of darkness, I had snuck into a friend's front yard with some mischievous girlfriends carrying fifty brightly coloured bars—the huge, oversized ones. We secured them throughout the beautiful trees growing around the front of the house... as an early birthday surprise, of course. We had an awful lot of fun hanging them up in the dark while imagining her reaction the next morning.

Chuckling from the memory, I decided that it would be better to ask for help. It was only a bra, for goodness sake. I unplugged the IV from the wall and quickly made my way to the nurses' station, rolling the IV pole on its noisy, wobbly wheels.

I tried to keep a small remnant of my dignity as I approached, carefully holding the hidden bra in my IV fist so no one would recognize what was in my hand. Looking as nonchalant as possible, I walked up to the first nurse I came across.

I felt like a little kid getting caught with her hand in the cookie jar!

"I have a slight dilemma," I began, "and I wonder if you could help me."

No words were necessary as I slowly opened my hand to display the neatly folded bra in my unclenched fist.

"I can't get it off because I'm attached to this," I added a few moments later, gently shaking the IV pole for added emphasis.

She looked down at the contents of my hand, then at the IV pole, then back up into my eyes. She started chuckling. Humour won over embarrassment and I joined in the laughter.

With quick efficiency, she helped me temporarily unplug from the IV tube, allowing me to slide the bra off my arm and patiently wait while she plugged me back in. With a smile and thank you, I then nonchalantly shoved the bra under my armpit and rolled back to my room.

Even when we're experiencing difficult situations, we can still find humour along the way, lightening the moment. More often than not, it'll lift our spirits and bring us much-needed glimmer of hope.

Journalling. I have found that writing helps build resilience. Many resources are available to help us cultivate a way of writing that fosters reflection and the release of unhelpful ideas to help us gain new insight and meaning.

One I have mentioned before was developed by Dr. James Pennebaker. His intentional process of expressive writing differs from normal journalling and can help produce new insights.

Some of our stories can be processed easily on our own, but other times we need to reach out for professional help because each person's experiences are different. It's not uncommon to go through painful or traumatic times in our lives when only a qualified professional can help us process our experiences in safe ways.

When I'm facing difficulties, I know that I must journal to create necessary margin. Then there are other times when writing is the last thing I want to do, and sometimes just talking it through with a trusted person helps create a bit of space in my head to begin writing. It will be different for everyone and will depend upon circumstances.

It's important to ask for help when needed.

Having fun. Play is important; moving our bodies is important. I've found that when I include fun and community into my week, I feel better and even more hopeful, because it helps me find pleasure, connection, and laughter.

It's normal to feel a little awkward when first meeting someone after a crisis, but given that we all suffer, and that our friends typically love us, being in community can be life-giving. Solitude is sometimes necessary, but isolation isn't helpful in the long run.

After having had a busy life managing kids, ongoing education, and a career, I had allowed much of my community to grow from these environments. Although my relationships were good, they often lacked intimacy.

As I inched closer to retirement, I knew I needed to deepen and enrich my community. I have always found city life to be isolating and have longed for a slower pace of life and to forge deep connections with others. I grew up in a small town on the south shore of Montreal where the culture was all about community. I longed to belong to such a rich community again.

Deciding to do something about it, I started a few groups. First, it was a women's book club, then a mixed games night—board games or pickleball. From these activities grew connections with others who enjoyed the same kinds of outings as my husband and me—specifically skiing, walking, camping, and kayaking.

I also invited some women to share regular online coffee times early on during the pandemic. This group has grown into a cherished group of special women who focus on personal formation and spiritual growth. Our friendships have expanded, life has happened for everyone, and our mutual appreciation and love has blossomed.

Instead of me wishing for community, I decided to create it and make the invitations. I'm glad I did. I'm now surrounded by a rich and beautiful community filled with diverse people of all ages—and it's life-giving to my soul.

Examen prayer. Saint Ignatius of Loyola, during the fifteenth century, developed a type of simple prayer called the Examen. It's a way of prayerfully reflecting on God's presence throughout our day and seeking guidance for our tomorrow. Often a prayer for day's end, it can be spoken midday as well.

The Examen includes prayerful consideration of how God's grace has been shown to us throughout the day, and how the circumstances of our day have affected us and may still be affecting us. It gives us a chance to consider our responses from the day and remember to respond with a heart of thankfulness as God changes and grows us through the process.

Upon completing the review of our day, the prayer shifts and looks forward to the next day. We can then ask God to show us how to prepare for tomorrow and consider how circumstances might sidetrack us from our purpose or calling. It ends with us asking God to give us what we need to be successful in the day ahead.

The Examen prayer helps us remember to think about God. It moves us from focusing on ourselves to focusing on Him, His ways, and how He might want to grow and transform us.

Cultivating a heart of gratitude. I have spoken about gratefulness previously and how it can help us cultivate faith-filled optimism. I've also written about the dangers of toxic positivity. So I'll be brief here, but the subject is important enough to turn into a regular practice.

Our inner life is so important and can impact every part of us, so being aware of our inner dialogue is important—because our words and thoughts are important.

It's hard to be grateful when things go wrong, and more often than not it's difficult to see anything good about a crisis or suffering while we're in the middle of it. It consumes the full space of our mind and heart.

Finding things to be thankful for helps builds resilience as long as we can be authentic without dismissing the challenges we face. Otherwise superficial types of gratitude aren't much different than toxic positivity. Forcing or faking gratitude doesn't help, either, because it can make us feel shame or guilt when we aren't yet ready to express gratitude.

Consider this: maybe gratitude isn't for ourselves, but for our understanding of who God is. How can we develop a heart of gratitude or rejoice for His goodness and steadfast love? We may be in crisis, but we need not be in despair because we have a source of hope to cling to—hope in God's goodness and His promises of the future. This can produce true thankfulness within us throughout the day.

Cultivating gratitude helps us remember to see good in the midst of challenges. It helps us learn to enjoy what we have right now despite our circumstances and limitations. It helps build space to grieve our losses and lament our challenges from a perspective of hope.

By cultivating this hope-filled gratitude, which is a type of rejoicing, we become more resilient. In this way, we may find that we can better value our relationships, cherish our time together (even if it's only online), or impart a kind word, smile, or chuckle.

Gratitude is contagious. When others catch our attitude of gratitude, it's most often reflected back toward us—which makes us even more grateful. Who knew that practicing gratitude would help us feel more gratitude!

Gratitude helps. It brings healing and cultivates hope. And it's a good practice to add to our soul care toolkit to help build resilience.

Try Your Own Soul Care Practices

As you explore your own ways of cultivating wholeness—mind, body, and spirit—may your hearts be filled with strength, great peace, God's steadfast love for you, and hope. I pray that you use this as an opportunity to try your own practices and discover new and different ways to care for your soul.

A Final Word

THIS BOOK IS A gift from my heart to yours. It's an integration of all of me. These insights have been, and still are, instrumental in moving me from a place of just surviving to thriving.

When we're faced with the unimaginable, we're often at a loss to understand how to cope in helpful ways. Although we can't always predict or change our circumstances, we must choose to look at the circumstances and come up with new approaches to deal with them. Our approach to dealing with crises can make a significant difference in what it means to choose to live well despite our circumstances.

There is no one-size-fits-all approach to walking through cancer, suffering, or grief. Each person's story is different and important. What helped me most was remembering what is true. Not a day went by when I didn't have to remind myself about what I believe. On the days when I forgot, God always brought me someone to help me remember.

Through the process of receiving such reminders, releasing unhelpful thinking, and embracing the remembering, I was able to remain open just enough to face the difficult twists and turns in my life.

I reminded myself that:

- Cancer and other health conditions often bring loss and unwanted changes. This makes it hard for us to see how our future could be good. But we can hope for good to come out of it. Look for and hang on to hope.

- Risk factors aren't the same as the actual causes of cancer. Blame and shame aren't helpful in healing.
- Comparison isn't helpful. No one's cancer is worse than another's; each experience is difficult.
- Grief is a silent partner of cancer, yet we can uncover some of our deepest longings as we process it.
- Asking for help when needed is a sign of courage.
- Labels are unhelpful. We aren't our health conditions; we aren't victims.
- We're more than good enough just as we are because of Whose we are!
- We're stronger together. Wisely choose an inner circle of support.
- We aren't ever alone. God promises to always walk with us.
- Practice presence and curiosity. Look for good. By doing so, we'll see more good in and around us.
- Cultivate patience. Deep healing is a slow process toward wholeness.
- Practice self-care and soul care. It's important to take the time needed to heal, inside and out.
- God's original design is for us is to be whole!

This book outlines portions of my story so far. Though I know yours is different than mine, deep down we aren't so very different—because we all face suffering in life.

If reading this book has challenged you, brought insight, or helped you to embrace even one new idea about wholeness, like how we're all designed to be whole, or if it's helped you embrace your belovedness in new ways, or if it's encouraged you to welcome a new understanding of what it means to embrace life and embrace hope, then I'm deeply grateful. We are stronger together.

If you want to stay in touch or hear more about hope, there are several options to stay connected:
- **Website:** www.hopeblooming.ca (Be sure to sign up for the monthly newsletter.)
- **Instagram:** www.instagram.com/hope.blooming
- **Facebook:** www.facebook.com/AtHopeBlooming

Acknowledgements

THIS BOOK EXISTS SOLELY because of the many sojourners who cheer me on. Without each one of them, this book would not be possible. Thank you to every one of you—you are my special community.

I must first thank my incredible husband. Thank you for your faithfulness as my beloved partner of forty-three years. When couples meet in their teens, special bonds are formed. In many ways, much of your heart is in this book too. I wouldn't want to do life with anyone else. Thank you for being my sounding board, for your countless hours of listening, and for reflecting and sharing your wisdom and insight. Thank you for your superpower of patience and steadfast love for me as I have recovered from treatment. I love you more than words can express.

I must also thank my four amazing kids, who have always cheered me on and kept checking in. And I also acknowledge my four charming grandchildren, who fill me with absolute delight and a strong will to live long and see them grow up. You all instill joy and hope in me, teaching me how precious time is when we spend it with one another. You are part of my heart and I love you dearly.

Thank you to my three siblings and their spouses—for your love, check-ins, and prayers from far. To my brother and sister-in-law, who live nearby, your love and kindness will always be cherished. Your consistent check-ins, talks, walks, visits, and thoughtfulness have been instrumental in my healing. Thank you. I love you all.

I also thank my friends, those who are in my inner circle and who warm my heart and make life a joy simply because of who you are and how you are in this world. Thank you for the walks, the talks, the shenanigans, and the meals we've shared together. Thank you for lovingly accepting the new me. My world is a better place because of you.

To my dear friend of thirty years, now gone to be with the Lord, thank you for your steadfast spirit and unwavering grasp of hope in your own battle with cancer, which continues to inspire me. Your absence has left a big void in many people's lives, especially those who loved and knew you. It was a privilege to call you a friend.

A special thanks to my pastor, his wife, and the church's pastoral team and support staff. Thank you for praying for me and for mobilizing leaders to faithfully pray for me.

Thank you to my prayer warriors, friends, and family for consistently encouraging me through texts and messages while in hospital. Thank you for your faithfulness. You were a much-needed lifeline for me during a time I shall never forget, and without you I never could have recovered as well as I have. Thank you for standing in the gap. You each know who you are.

To my surgeons, thank you for your faithful ongoing care, kindness, and humour which help me to look forward to my follow-up appointments. Without you and your stellar team of residents, not to mention your tireless commitment to helping cancer patients survive, I wouldn't be here today and would not be doing as well as I am. And a deep thanks to the two special surgeons for their ongoing care. You two gentlemen are my heroes.

To all my other doctors, dentists, and support professionals, thank you for providing ongoing care, exercise classes, and support for me during the early months and throughout all the other conditions and issues that cropped up as I recovered, and for all your efforts in helping me to stay healthy and strong.

A very special thanks to the hospital and cancer centre nurses, aides, occupational therapists, respiratory therapists, psychologists, social workers, and nutritionists, oncologists, oncology nurse-practitioners, radiation technicians, speech therapists, physiotherapists, dentists, hygienists, psychosocial counsellors, and other support staff who have assisted me. You have played roles facilitating my healing. To this amazing team, I owe great thanks to you for caring for me while I was in the hospital.

I thank my writing coach for your ability to cheer me on while also making important, wise suggestions to challenge my writing—and most of all, for helping me find my voice. I think I finally found it! Thank you!

To my endorsers, you guys are heroes and leaders with whom I am privileged to share life, near and afar. I appreciate your steadfastness and perseverance in providing your feedback. Thank you for your love, faithful friendship, and ongoing encouragement.

Many others have sent me words of encouragement and love, and they are too numerous to mention. Each has fuelled me to keep writing and each holds a special place in my heart: my ministry colleagues, counselling colleagues, book club friends, fellow artists, and fellow writers. You have built strength into me in some way through your words, prayers, and support. Thank you for walking with me and encouraging me to find true hope, taking one step at a time toward wholeness. These experiences have helped me learn, when facing my own unimaginable crisis, to dig deep, draw close to God, draw close to safe community, and find ways to embrace my new normal.

I must also thank my readers. Thank you for reading my story. I hope it has made you curious about your own story in new ways and inspired you to find new ways to embrace hope and wholeness in it.

And finally, I offer a special thank you for supporting cancer research and/or cancer support programs for cancer patients and families.

About the Author

FERN E.M. BUSZOWSKI, A RECENT oral cancer survivor, counsellor, and retired pastor of counselling and soul care, has dedicated her life to empowering others to grow, develop, and find hope. With two master's degrees, one in ministry and leadership and the other in counselling, she uniquely weaves concepts and practices from different fields to help others learn to cultivate sacred space for their souls.

She served most of her career giving back to her community in non-profit, educational, and charity settings. Her unique combination of education has equipped her to draw from the best of two worlds to provide holistic counselling and soul care for many individuals, groups, and couples seeking healing, wholeness, and growth.

Professionally, Fern has written and designed training programs and resources, *Soul Care Companioning*, *Unstuck*, and *Sojourning*, and developed peer-led programs to train leaders who wish to journey alongside those seeking healing and wholeness. She has also spent time equipping and developing her own teams of volunteer lay leaders to provide care and compassionate support in various settings. She has provided coaching, team-building workshops, and coach training in local and international settings for charity-based leaders. These training programs have concentrated on enhancing team dynamics, communication, and collaboration in international settings with remote teams.

Her extensive experience with personality assessments and tools (such as EQ-I 2.0, Birkman, GRIP-Birkman, and Myers Briggs I/II) have helped her provide training for undergraduate behavioural science students who are preparing for practicum placements.

She now spends much of her free time being a grandma to her four delightful grandchildren, writing, painting, connecting with friends, and spending time outdoors. This includes training her dog Bailey, who aspires to be a therapy visitation dog encouraging others.

Fern E.M. Buszowski lives with her husband Steve in the foothills of Alberta with their ginger-coloured mini-Australian labradoodle. They have two grown married daughters and two sons-in-law.

Endnotes

[1] Henri Nouwen, With Open Hands (Notre Dame, IN: Ave Maria Press, 2006), 75–76.

[2] "Oral and Oropharyngeal Cancer: Statistics," Cancer.net. March 2022 (https://www.cancer.net/cancer-types/oral-and-oropharyngeal-cancer/statistics).

[3] C.S. Lewis, "First and Second Things," *God in the Dock* (Grand Rapids, MI: William B. Eerdmans Publishing Co., 1970), 278–280.

[4] Sean Campbell, "Equip Winter 2022, Sean Campbell," YouTube. March 10, 2022 (https://www.youtube.com/watch?v=o9vBqHeaZNs).

[5] Curt Thompson, Facebook. January 11, 2022 (https://www.facebook.com/photo.php?fbid=278171720965398&set=pb.100063177163175.-2207520000.&type=3).

[6] David Wallin, Attachment in Psychotherapy (New York, NY: The Guilford Press, 2007), 12.

[7] David Benner, Surrender to Love: Discovering the Heart of Christian Spirituality (Downers Grove, IL: InterVarsity Press, 2003), 17.

[8] Richard Rhor, Falling Upward: A Spirituality for the Two Halves of Life (San Francisco, CA: Jossy-Bass, 2011), 146.

[9] Ibid.

[10] Fern E.M. Buszowski, UNSTUCK (Calgary, AB: First Alliance Church, 2016). These questions have been slightly modified from the 2016 publication.

[11] Brené Brown, The Gifts of Imperfection: Let Go of Who You Think You're Supposed to Be and Embrace Who You Are (Center City, MN: Hazelden, 2010), ix).

[12] Ann Voskamp, Facebook. October 1, 2020 (https://www.facebook.com/AnnVoskamp/photos/a.369461463066034/3901731746505637).

[13] James W. Pennebaker and John F. Evans, Expressive Writing: Words that Heal (Enumclaw, WA: Idyll Arbour, Inc., 2014).

[14] Curt Thompson, MD Facebook. March 31, 2022 (https://www.facebook.com/CurtThompsonMD/posts/pfbid029hzhSaANJtqhJ5iHtpE2pN5RuYncYYw5iEWs6bGRvhnH7mCyduzWf3jfYigEkXGTl).

[15] Dan Allender, To Be Told: God Invites You to Coauthor Your Future (Colorado Springs, CO: Waterbrook Press, 2005), 3.

[16] C.S. Lewis, The Last Battle (New York, NY: Harper Collins Children's Books, 1994), 25. First published in 1956.

[17] "Persevere," Online Etymology Dictionary. Date of access: September 9, 2022 (https://www.etymonline.com/word/persevere#etymonline_v_12743).

[18] "Continue," Online Etymology Dictionary. Date of access: December 11, 2022 (https://www.etymonline.com/search?q=continue).

[19] C.S. Lewis, A Grief Observed: Reader's Edition (London, UK: Faber and Faber, Ltd., 2014), 196. First published in 1961.

[20] Alan Wolfelt, "Grief," Center for Loss and Transition. Date of access: September 12, 2022 (https://www.centerforloss.com/grief).

[21] Margery Williams, The Velveteen Rabbit (New York, NY: Doubleday, 1922), 5.

[22] Ibid., 5-8.

[23] Brené Brown, Connections: A 12-Session Psychoeducational Shame-Resilience Curriculum (Minneapolis, MN: Hazelden Publishing, 2009).

[24] Ibid., 42.

[25] Meg Apperson, "From Broken to Beautiful: When You Need to Believe There Is a Plan for Your Pain," Ann Voskamp. Date of access: September 12, 2022 (https://annvoskamp.com/2020/10/from-broken-to-beautiful-when-you-need-to-believe-theres-a-plan-for-your-pain).

[26] Timothy Keller, Walking with God through Pain and Suffering (New York, NY: Penguin Group, 2013), 190–191.

[27] Ibid., 13.

[28] John Ortberg, Soul Keeping: Caring for the Most Important Part of You (Grand Rapids, MI: Zondervan, 2014), 23. Quoting Dallas Willard.

[29] "Resilient," Online Etymology Dictionary. Date of access: October 6, 2022 (https://www.etymonline.com/search?q=resilient).

[30] Thich Truong, Instagram. Date of access: December 15, 2022 (https://www.instagram.com/p/CmNSQ2-P4Jw).

[31] John Piper, "What Is Hope?" Desiring God. April 1986 (https://www.desiringgod.org/messages/what-is-hope).

[32] John Swinton, Finding Jesus in the Storm: The Spiritual Lies of Christians with Mental Health Challenges (Grand Rapids, MI: William B. Eerdmans Publishing Co., 2020), 205–206.

[33] "Hope," Online Etymology Dictionary. Date of access: November 8, 2022 (https://www.etymonline.com/word/hope).

[34] Ronne Rock, Facebook. May 27, 2022 (https://www.facebook.com/RonneRockWrites/photos/a.823818571012338/5324798420914308).